Lynda AOUDIA

Elastography of breast masses

Lynda AOUDIA

Elastography of breast masses

Elastography performance in breast mass characterization

ScienciaScripts

Imprint
Any brand names and product names mentioned in this book are subject to trademark, brand or patent protection and are trademarks or registered trademarks of their respective holders. The use of brand names, product names, common names, trade names, product descriptions etc. even without a particular marking in this work is in no way to be construed to mean that such names may be regarded as unrestricted in respect of trademark and brand protection legislation and could thus be used by anyone.

Cover image: www.ingimage.com

This book is a translation from the original published under ISBN 978-613-8-40264-0.

Publisher:
Sciencia Scripts
is a trademark of
Dodo Books Indian Ocean Ltd. and OmniScriptum S.R.L publishing group

120 High Road, East Finchley, London, N2 9ED, United Kingdom
Str. Armeneasca 28/1, office 1, Chisinau MD-2012, Republic of Moldova, Europe
Managing Directors: Ieva Konstantinova, Victoria Ursu
info@omniscriptum.com

Printed at: see last page
ISBN: 978-620-8-57063-7

Contents

I dedicate this work

To my very eher father, you surrounded me with attention, instilled in me the noble values of life and the importance of integrity, taught me the art of a job well done, and the sense of responsibility, you were a great support throughout my studies, thank you for everything you did and still do for me, may God keep you and grant you a long life.

To my very dear Mother, who without her presence, her patience and her continuous support, especially at the hardest times, when Ton doubted everything, this work would never have seen the light of day. I offer this work especially to her, saying thank you, may the Lord grant you a long life.

My dear sister Nabila, and her adorable son Lyna, thank you for your precious support.

To the memory of my dear sister Siham, we will always keep you in our hearts and you were a model courage and success right up to the end. To your adorable children Rafik and Ania, may God keep them.

To my dear brothers Abd El Fateh and Mohamed Amine, thank you for all your help and encouragement throughout the preparation of this work.

To my dear friends, Wahiba and Assia, for their support and presence, I say thank you from the bottom of my heart.

To all those who have passed through my life and left a pleasant memory.

Introduction

Today, breast imaging enables sub-clinical lesions to be detected and charactcrised. Detection is still based on mammography, which is the reference examination for breast cancer screening and remains the only technique capable of detecting certain lesions such as microcalcifications.

However, while the overall sensitivity of mammography is good (70-90%) [Ió], it is much lower in patients with dense breasts (30-48%), in whom cancers may be masked by superimposed glandular tissue [7-8]. In these patients, ultrasound is recommended to detect cancers that are hidden by mammography [9]. Ultrasound is also indicated, as a first-line procedure or in addition to mammography, to assess the degree of suspicion of an abnormality. When a breast abnormality is detected on imaging, it needs to be characterised in order to assess the risk it being cancer.

Classically, this assessment is based on morphological criteria (shape, contours, orientation in relation to the skin, interface, echogenicity, posterior acoustic signs), according to which abnormalities are classified in one of the five categories of the American College of Radiology (ACR) Bf-RADS (Breast fmaging- Reporting and Data System) lexicon, depending on the degree of suspicion [10]. This classification, based on the degree of risk of cancer, enables appropriate management to be proposed.

Category 1 corresponds to the absence of abnormality. Certain anomalies present a morphological aspect typical of benignity, classified as Bf-RADS 2 with a PPV = 0%, or typical of malignancy, classified as Bf-RADS 5, PPV of cancer > 95%. For other anomalies, most probably benign, classified as Bf- RADS 3 with a VPP of cancer < 2%, simple surveillance is indicated. In some cases, the morphological criteria usually seen on ultrasound are not sufficient to determine whether a lesion is benign or malignant, a so-called "undetermined lesion", often classified as Bf-RADS 4, with a cancer PPV of between 2 and 95%, and it is therefore necessary to propose a biopsy, which in most cases corresponds to benign lesions that could only be checked by non-invasive imaging. The consequences of these undetermined lesions are not trivial, as there are complications and potential adverse effects associated with any percutaneous invasive procedure, including unnecessary anxiety, infection, haematoma, etc[ll].

In ultrasound, it is estimated that 47% to 84% of unnecessary biopsies are carried out for benign lesions, which could be avoided [12-18]. On the other hand, some cancers, including the most aggressive high-grade cancers, may paradoxically have morphological features suggestive of benignity, such as an oval shape and/or circumscribed contours [19], which may be wrongly considered reassuring.

MRI is a very good tool for abnormalities thanks to its high sensitivity, but its low specificity means that it is of little use in characterising breast lesions, and so does not reduce the number of negative biopsies of abnormalities that are not detected by ultrasound [20, 21].

The development of new additional parameters, different from the usual morphological parameters, is therefore necessary to assess the nature of the lesion more reliably. In ultrasound, new imaging tools have been developed in recent years, such as elastography. Elastography, a technique developed in the late 90s, is now routinely available on new ultrasound scanners. This technique makes it possible to assess the hardness or elasticity of tissues, or their relative displacements, in order to produce an image of elasticity or deformation, information which has historically been assessed by palpation and which constitutes an important element in clinical diagnosis. However, the elasticity assessed by clinical examination depends on the operator, the size and location (depth) of the lesion and the structure of the breast.

Breast elastography uses two distinct modes: free-hand elastography and shear-wave elastography. Classically, malignant breast lesions are more rigid than benign lesions. This new ultrasound parameter is added to the morphological and vascularisation criteria in the diagnostic approach to breast lesions. In our study, we propose to evaluate the contribution of elastography to the characterisation of benign and malignant breast lesions.

CHAPTER 1

Literature and issues

1. Literature data

1.1. Epidemiology

Breast cancer is the most common cancer in women worldwide, with an estimated 2.2 million new cases diagnosed in 2020 (24.5% of all cancers), and it remains the leading cause of cancer death in women worldwide [22].
Data from Algerian registries show an incidence of 70 per 100,000 women, i.e. 10,000 new cases per year [23].
In Algeria, the average age of onset of this cancer in women is 49, i.e. 10 to 15 years younger than in the Western population, according to the various Algerian registries [24-27].
Its incidence has increased steadily over the last few decades, rising in 20 years from an overall incidence of 100 per 100,000 population to 120 per 100,000 population [28]. In women, breast cancer ranks first in terms of incidence of new cases in the 3 main Algerian registries [24-26]. Its adjusted standardised incidence (ASA) is 21.6, 17.03 and 34.49 per 100,000 women for the Algiers, Sétif and Oran registries, respectively. The change between 1986 and 2005 is marked by a variation in l'fSA from 10.4 per 100,000 women for the period 1986-1989, to 17 per 100,000 women for the period 1993-1997 and 14.2 per 100,000 women for the period 2001-2005 [29].
In Algeria, the mortality rate is 18.5 per 100,000 women, with an estimated 4,116 deaths per year [22].

1.2. Ultrasound

Ultrasound is an accessible, non-irradiating and inexpensive imaging technique. It may be indicated as a complement to mammography, to improve lesion detection, particularly in dense breasts [30], to characterise lesions, in particular to differentiate solid lesions from cystic lesions, and to take samples.
Breast ultrasound is performed with a high-frequency probe, usually between 9 and 5 MHz, which provides both good contrast and good spatial resolution [31].1 There are several ultrasound modes.

1.2.1. Ultrasound techniques

1.2.1.1. The B mode

This is the first technique performed during breast ultrasound. Ultrasound waves are emitted and collected by the probe, at the same frequency, in a single direction. They are combined to create a 2D image of the breast on a greyscale [32]. This technique allows structures to be differentiated on the basis of the acoustic and mechanical properties of the tissue. This B mode has some weaknesses, including inconsistent optimal resolution and artefacts that can degrade image quality [33].

1.2.1.2. Harmonic mode

This is linked to the non-linear behaviour of breast tissue in relation to ultrasound. As the ultrasound wave propagates through breast tissue, it progressive distortion of the shape of the ultrasound pulse, creating harmonic frequencies which are multiples of the emission frequency [34-36]. Once the initial signal has been filtered, the harmonic signal is used for image reconstruction. This technique makes it possible to improve the contrast of ultrasound images, particularly in the case of "thick-content" cysts or complicated cysts, which in B mode show internal echoes whereas in harmonic mode appear anechoic [37].

1.2.1.3. Compound mode

There are two types of composite, frequency composite (several different ultrasound emission frequencies are used to reconstruct the final image), and spatial composite (several ultrasound emission angles are used and combined into a single composite image). This technique makes it possible to limit artefacts, improve analysis of lesion contours, better define the internal echostructure of masses and detect small lesions [38]. It also allows better detection of intra-lesional calcifications [39]. On the other hand, posterior ultrasound changes are attenuated [40].

1.2.1.4. Colour Doppler mode

It enables tumour angiogenesis to be detected. Malignant lesions are generally more vascularised than benign lesions, with an abnormal, irregular appearance of the vessels. Detection and analysis of spectrum of these vessels requires a probe of at least 10 MHz and a rigorous ultrasound technique (adjustment of the focal length, reduction of the overall gain, adaptation of the size of the doppler box, filtering to a minimum of 10 in order analyse the low frequencies, no pressure on the breast to avoid obliteration of the small vessels) [41,42].

Energy Doppler has a better sensitivity to slow flows but is more sensitive to artefacts [43]. Doppler can be used to analyse hypoechoic lesions which pose a "cystic or solid" problem. The presence of vascularisation in an echogenic lesion indicates that the lesion is tissue. On the other hand, the absence of vascularisation does not rule out the presence of a tissue portion [32]. There is considerable overlap in Doppler mapping between benign and malignant lesions [32, 44], which does not improve the specificity of ultrasound for solid masses.

1.3. Lesion characterisation on ultrasound 1.3.1. Cystic versus solid lesion

Ultrasound can improve the specificity of mammography, particularly for distinguishing cystic and solid lesions. When all the criteria for a simple cyst are present, i.e. anechoic lesion, circumscribed, with posterior enhancement, no solid component and no Doppler signal, the accuracy of ultrasound is 96 to 100% [12].

A complicated cyst is a remodelled cyst with a thick protein or haemorrhagic content. Colour Doppler can help us to differentiate a cyst with thick contents from a solid lesion. According to Berg et al (ACRIN Study 6666) [45], only 12% of complicated cysts reported correspond to solid lesions with a malignancy rate of 0.42%; these authors classify these lesions as BI-RADS 3 and recommend monitoring at 6 months. In the event of a change in size of more than 20% of the diameter in 6 months, sampling for diagnostic purposes was indicated [40, 46].

Finally, atypical cysts, known as complex cystic masses, are cysts with a solid portion; in 75% of cases, these are benign papilloma-type lesions, and in 20% of cases the lesions are malignant. These complex cystic masses are considered suspicious, classified as Bi-RADS 4, and sampling is indicated [47].

1.3.1. Benign versus malignant solid lesions

Stavros [12] was the first to describe specific ultrasound criteria for benign and malignant masses. Malignant masses were often associated with spiculated, irregular or microlobulated contours, a strongly hypoechoic echostructure and posterior attenuation. In this study, these criteria had an excellent sensitivity of 98.4%, a specificity of 67.8% and a negative predictive value of 99.5%. Some criteria, such as shape and contours had a higher predictive value than others, e.g. echostructure and posterior acoustic effect. The combination of these characteristics allows a good diagnostic orientation (Cf. Appendix 1) [48, 49]. The absence of malignancy criteria is correlated with an excellent negative predictive value.

Complexity seems to persist regarding the low specificity of undetermined or suspect criteria, which are often found in benign lesions.

1.3.2. Limits

1.3.2.1. Inter-observer variability

The operator-dependent nature of ultrasound is one of the major drawbacks of the examination [50, 51]. It is this inter-observer variability in the description and assessment of solid masses on ultrasound that has led to the need to standardise the terminology used in mammary ultrasound, and is at the origin of the ultrasound glossary in the 4th edition of BI-RADS® [51].

1.3.2.2. Variability in relation to the BI-RADS lexicon

[52,53].

With regard to the BI-RADS lexicon, studies have shown high inter-observer agreement for lesional calcifications, moderate to high agreement for the assessment of shape, orientation and interface, and moderate agreement for posterior acoustic effects.

However, agreement was poor for the assessment of lesion contours and echogenicity. The inter-observer variations observed in the assessment of lesion contours mainly related to the different descriptors used for non-circumscribed lesions (microlobulated, irregular, angular, spiculated). However, whatever the terminology used for non-circumscribed lesions, in all cases this is a criterion of malignancy and therefore the final assessment is not affected [54]. Lesion echogenicity, however, is not considered to be a very useful criterion for differentiating benign and malignant masses [12].

1.3.2.3. Variability in relation to the final BIRADS devaluation category

With regard to the analysis of inter-observer variability of the final BIRADS, studies have shown discordant results, ranging from high inter-observer agreement for the Lee study [55], moderate for Park et al [56] and Berg et al [57], and low for the Lazarus study [52], especially for BI-RADS 4.

1.3.2.4. Low specificity of ultrasound

Ultrasound is a very sensitive examination, but has low specificity. Specificity varies between 45 and 93% [58] depending on the appearance of the lesions, the type of equipment and the radiologist's experience.

1.4. Elastography

In Hippocratic medicine, palpation is a key part of the clinical examination. It is the first step in screening for a number of cancers. When a nodule is found in the breast, thyroid, prostate, etc., palpation tries to assess its hardness. Generally speaking, lesions that are hard, irregular and fixed to the deep surface are more likely to be malignant, whereas lesions that are soft, well defined and mobile in relation to the deep surface are more likely to be benign. In reality, palpation provides a subjective assessment of tissue rigidity, i.e. its Young's modulus. However, it has its limitations in small or deep-seated tumours.

Elastography is a non-invasive technique used in conjunction with ultrasound to qualitatively, semi-quantitatively or quantitatively assess the deformability of lesions subjected to stress [59-61]. The image obtained is translated into an elastogram. This technique was developed to improve the specificity of B-mode breast ultrasound, by adding compressibility and lesion hardness to the morphological criteria for lesions .

The idea of using ultrasound to assess the deformability of tissue dates back to 1983, when A. Eisenscher [62] described a technique known as echoseismography, which used the TM mode. In 1991, J. Ophir gave the technique the name of elastography [61]. The first in vivo studies date back to the mid-1990s [63].

Elastography is currently the subject of a great deal of research and publication in the field of breast imaging [64-66], but is also making progress in the imaging of other organs such as the thyroid, liver and prostate [67].

1.4.1. Physical principle

We must always go back to definitions:

Hardness is the ability of a material to withstand stress.

Rigidity is the degree of elastic deformation of the material under this stress.

Elasticity is the ability of a material to return to its initial shape when subjected to stress or mechanical oscillation.

A benign lesion is normally firmer than normal surrounding breast tissue but softer than a malignant lesion [68]. This notion is explained by the modulus of elasticity or Young's modulus.

Thomas Young (1773-1829) was a British physician and physicist who noticed that the ratio between the tensile stress applied to an isotropic homogeneous material and the resulting deformation, "relative elongation", is constant as long as the deformation remains moderate and the material's elastic limit is not reached. This constant is called Young's modulus or longitudinal modulus of elasticity.

If σ is stress, 8 is strain and E is Young's modulus, Hooke's law is: σ = E 8 (fig. 1). For the same stress, a material with a high modulus of elasticity (E) will undergo less deformation than a material with a lower modulus of elasticity (E). Young's modulus has a large dynamic range between different biological tissues, which makes it ideal for characterising different tissues [69]. In general, fatty tissue deforms more easily than fibrous or cancerous tissue and returns to its initial state more slowly than fat or muscle [70].

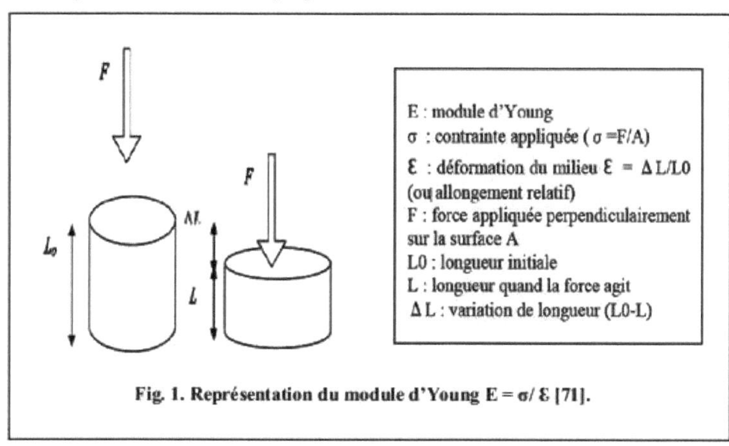

Fig. 1. Représentation du module d'Young E = σ/ Ɛ [71].

E: Young's modulus
σ: applied stress (σ =F/A)
£ deformation of the medium E = Δ L/LO (or| relative elongation)
F: force applied perpendicularly to the surface A
LO: initial length
L: length when the force acts
Δ L: variation in length (LO-L)

Fig. 1 Young's modulus E= σ/ E [71].

Young's modulus is expressed in terms of the compression modulus (K) and the shear modulus (μ) (fig. 2). In soft biological tissues, Young's modulus is the main reflection of the shear modulus:

E = 9 Kμ which can be simplified to 3 μ.

3 K+μ

Elastography, by using inter-correlation techniques between successive ultrasound images, makes it possible to monitor tissue deformation and produce a map tissue Young's modulus. It has been said that elastography is "computer-assisted palpation".

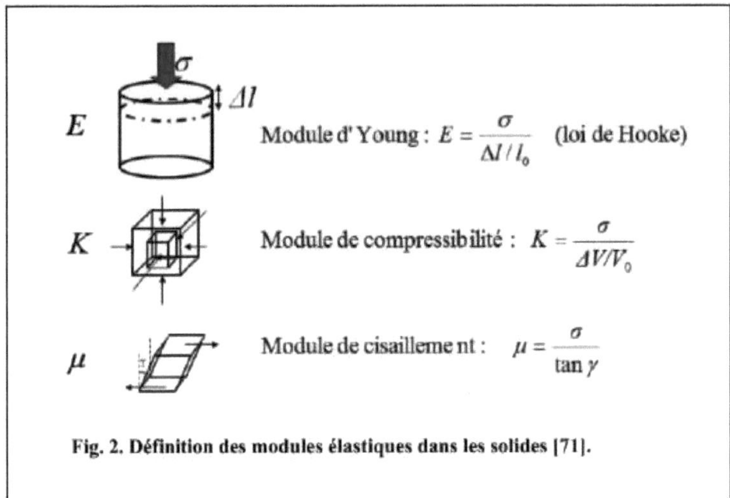

Fig. 2. Définition des modules élastiques dans les solides [71].

There are two basic types of deformation that an elastic solid can undergo: uniform compression (change of volume without change of shape) and sliding or shearing (change of shape without change of volume) (fig. 3).

Elastography is the coupling of a mechanical stress (which produces the strain) to a system for measuring tissue displacements [70].

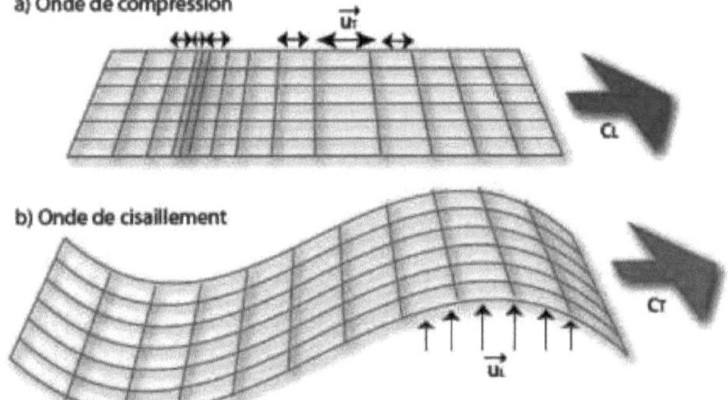

Fig. 3 Elementary deformation of an elastic solid. a) The compression wave (P) propagates through successive variations in the volume of the medium. The displacement of the medium u is parallel to its direction of propagation with a velocity CL. Ultrasound, used in echography, is a compressional wave. Sound is also a compression wave in the audible frequency range; b) the shear wave (S) propagates by successive movements perpendicular to the direction of propagation with a speed CT [72].

The mechanical load may be :

- Static: manual compression of the breast. Deformation occurs very slowly and is therefore quasi-static. Viscosity effects are not present and the material behaves like a pure solid [73].
- Dynamics: by setting up a continuous low-frequency vibration. Transient effects are not present and the waves can be considered to be in a stationary state [74]. The given non-zero frequency means that viscosity has to be taken into account and the stationary state leads to reflections which require the acquisition of 3D data, such as 3D ultrasound.
- Impulsive: mechanical excitation involves a mechanical shock with a fairly wide bandwidth. A set of waves propagating at different frequencies is emitted towards the object. This method requires very high temporal resolution to distinguish the different frequency components and is therefore typically used in ultrasound because of its real-time imaging [75, 76].

1.4.2. Elastography techniques [77-81]

Elastography is the ratio of stress to strain. All existing techniques are based on these three steps:

- application of an excitation to the tissue, resulting in a static or dynamic response involving longitudinal or shear elastic properties;
- imaging of disrupted tissue ;
- from the various images, determination of a parameter dependent on the type of excitation and the hardness of the tissue.

The different techniques are classified according to the action exerted on the tissues and are of two types in ultrasound:

- Static elastography (also known as relative, stress or strain elastography), which uses the Young's modulus (E) to visualise its deformation;
- measure its capacity to modify the speed of a wave passing through it: this is transitorient elastography (or Shear Waves), which uses the shear modulus (μ).

1.4.2.1. Static elastography or Strain Imaging

In the early 1990s, Ophir's team developed the first elastography technique [61]. The technique was tested on breast cancers with interesting results [82]. This method only allows a qualitative assessment of Young's modulus. The probe is manually compressed extempore and the displacement of the tissue before and after compression is then measured. It is used to assess the axial and lateral deformation of lesions under axial stress (Fig. 4) [83]. It is a simple and rapid method that requires a learning period.

This technique produces results:

- Qualitative aspects differ from one manufacturer to another.
- Semi-quantitative.

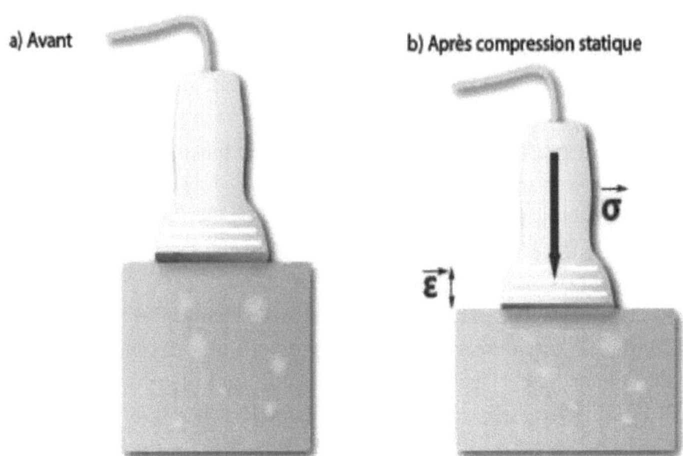

Fig. *4:* **Principle of static elastography.**

Static elastography reconstructs an elastogram by calculating the deformations due to static compression exerted by the operator through the ultrasound probe. [72].

1.4.2.1.1. Qualitative analysis

This is an evaluation of the elastogram, which differs depending on the manufacturer, either according to the grey scale or the colour scale. Static elastography analyses images of tissue subjected low-amplitude pressure-decompression movements. These images are acquired in real time and in colour and graded according to the Ueno and Itoh classification into five categories [84] (fig. 5) for the Hitachi model. Lesions 1 to 3 are considered benign and lesions 4 and 5 malignant.

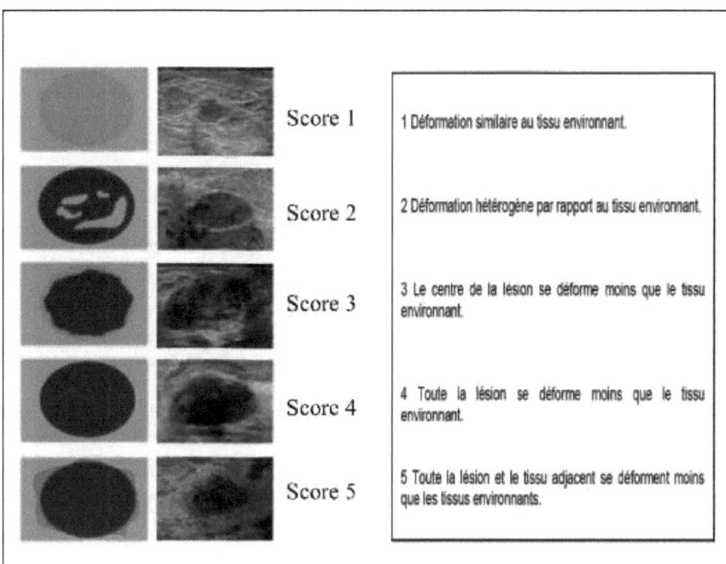

Fig. 5. Score de l'université de Tskukuba. Une échelle couleur de 1 à 5 est associée à un risque accru de malignité.

1.4.2.1.2. Quantitative analysis

a. Elasticity ratio

By calculating the Fat Lesion Ratio or Strain Ratio (FLR) [84]. The FLR is expressed as a standard deviation.

FLR = average speed of the surrounding fat / average speed of the lesion.

This measure quantifies the elasticity correlation between two regions of interest. The first region of interest delimits the lesion and the second is the reference region corresponding to the surrounding fat [85, 86]. This measurement is independent of the compression movement exerted by the radiologist (fig. 6).

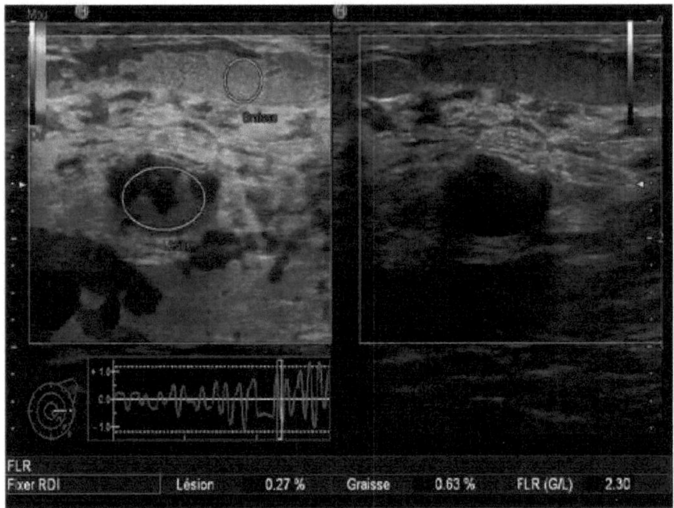

Fig. 6: Calculation of the elasticity ratio using static elastography. The first ROI (L) is traced in the lesion and the second ROI (G) is traced in the subcutaneous fat. The G/L ratio corresponds to the elasticity ratio, which in this example is calculated as 2.30.
Histology: fibroadenoma.

b. Size ratio

Assessment of the size ratio is the ratio of the size of the lesion on B-mode ultrasound and that on the elastographic image [87-90]. A benign lesion is usually more flexible done more deformable, observed often smaller in elastography than in B mode, while the size of malignant tumours on elastography is larger than that observed in B mode (fig. 7) [91].

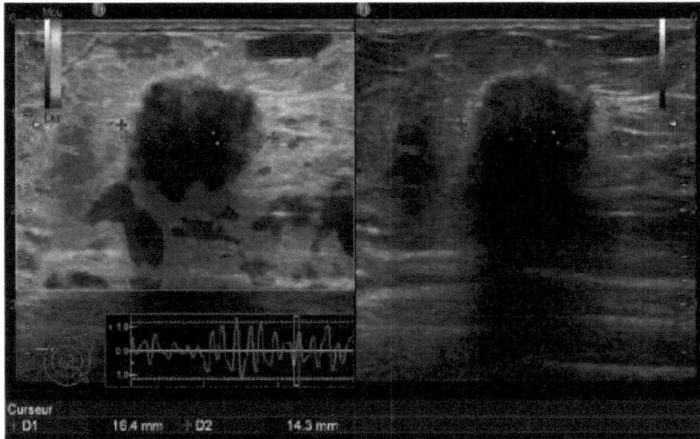

Fig. 7 Calculation of the size ratio in static elastography. The ratio of the longest axis of

the lesion measured on the elastographic image and the longest axis of the corresponding image measured on B-mode ultrasound. The size ratio in this example was calculated to be 1.15. Histology: NST infllrant carcinoma.

This technique has been studied objectively in a number of scientific studies using different devices, showing variable results with sensitivities of between 70.1% and 86.5% and specificities of between 84% and 95.7% [84, 92-96]. In a multicentre study involving nine centres and 442 lesions classified as Bi-RADS 3 and 4, the sensitivity was 68% and the specificity 90% [96]. According to the studies, when elastography is combined with B-mode ultrasound, an improvement in specificity is found [65, 97].

In the study by Thomas [97] of 108 lesions, 49 of which were malignant, specificity was increased but to a variable extent depending on the observer (+ 6.7 to 13.5%) compared with B-mode ultrasound.

1.4.2.2. Shear wave elastography

The Ondes et Acoustique laboratory at the École Supérieure de Physique et Chimie Industrielle in Paris has implemented transitorient elastography, coupling a prototype ultrasound image to a low-frequency mechanical vibration used on the body surface.

Several years of research have succeeded in detecting breast tumours in vivo using a prototype [99]. New advances in research have made it possible to replace the external vibrator with an ultrasound beam focused for a few hundred milliseconds (ms); this beam moves the tissue by a few tens of microns. The same ultrasound probe is now used to vibrate tissues at a distance and rapidly image their movements.

Shear wave elastography is a new elastography technique that records transverse displacements and shear wave propagation generated by focused ultrasound. Elasticity is directly related to propagation speed. Capturing and recording displacements involves acquiring several thousand images per second.

Three waves are involved in shear wave elastography (fig. 8):

- The initial wave, or ultrasound compression wave, is generated by the median zone of the probe, rhythmically, every 2 seconds, without operator intervention. It is an extremely fast wave (Bulk wave) (1550 m/s), which generates an ultrasound signal known as the "Mach signal".
- At a focal point, this wave will generate an acoustic radiation force which generates perpendicular waves which will progress tangentially across the skin. These shear waves are slower than the initial wave (1-10 m/s) and their speed is increased when they pass through a harder structure (fig. 9) [100].
- The third wave is the insonation beam, which makes it possible to record variations in speed and thus deduce μ, the shear modulus. Young's modulus E is 3 times the shear modulus, so can be used to assign a value to hardness in kPa [101].

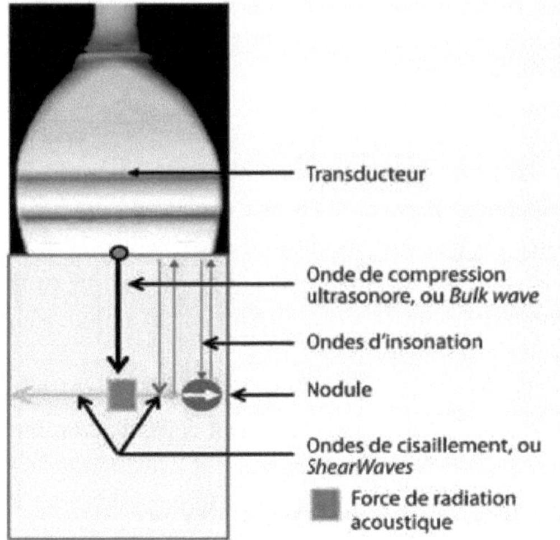

Transducer
Ultrasonic compression wave, or *Bulk wave*
Insonation waves
Nodule
Shear *waves*
Acoustic radiation force

Fig. 8: Shear wave elastography [101].

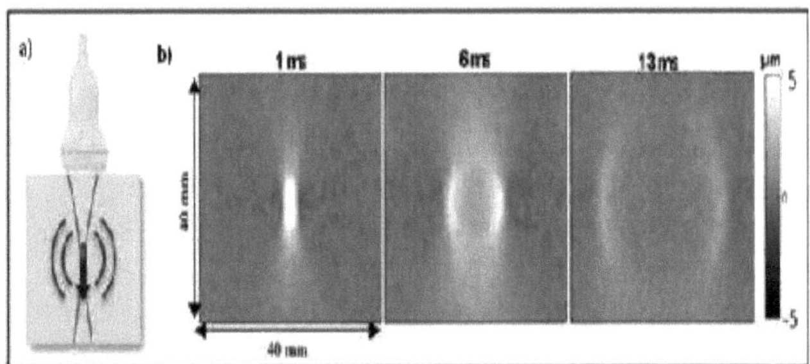

Fig. 9 Ultrasonic radiation force, (a) A radiation force can be applied to tissue by emitting a focused ultrasound shot using a conventional ultrasound probe. (b) Axial displacements induced by ultrasonic radiation force in an agar-gelatine gel. The ultrasound frequency is 4.3 MHz, the duration of the ultrasound shot is 100 ps [100].

This technique gives qualitative results in terms of colour scale and quantitative results. In the study by A. Athanasiou [102], malignant lesions had an elasticity of E= 170.1 +/- 42 kPa, while benign lesions had an elasticity of E= 53 +/- 19.8 kPa. For cysts, the elasticity was 0 kPa.

The advantage of this technique is its insensitivity to motion artefacts. There are two commercially available technologies for this recording, Supersonic Shear Imaging (SSI) and Acoustic Radiation Force Impulse (ARFI) [103].

1.4.2.2.1. Supersonic Shear Imaging technology

This system consists a beamformer that uses the radio frequency signal produce more than 5000 images per second and to record variations in the speed of the tangential wave. The hardness value of the structures crossed by the shear wave is given in real time [102, 104].

Thanks to an ultra-fast collection technique, the propagation of shear waves can be followed in real time. The source of vibration of the wave is "supersonic", making it possible to increase the speed of propagation of the shear waves and to focus them at the desired depth while reducing the acoustic energy used [104, 105] (fig. 10). In a medium containing a hard lesion, the shear wave is deformed and its speed is accelerated. Its displacement is closely linked to the viscoelastic properties of the tissue; a quantitative elasticity map is thus obtained (fig. 11).

The advantages of SWE elastography are that it can be performed during the ultrasound examination, that it is quantitative and that it is virtually insensitive to motion artefacts. In terms of risks, it has been shown that the acoustic intensity induced is below the levels defined by the Food and Drug Administration (510K standard) [104].

In one of the articles published by Evans et al [106], they found that this technique had a sensitivity of 95%, a specificity of 77%, a positive predictive value of 84% and a negative predictive value of 91%.

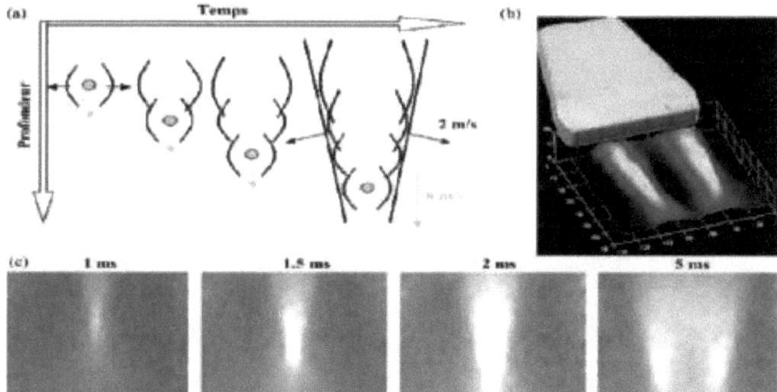

Fig. 10 Principle of shear wave elastography. (a) Principle of generating a shear source travelling at supersonic speed. lei, the source travels at 6 m/s compared with a shear wave speed of 2 m/s. (b) Three-dimensional representation of the micrometric displacements induced in the ultrasound imaging yoke. **(b)** Three-dimensional representation of the micrometric displacements induced in the ultrasound imaging yaw. **(c)** Axial displacements produced in supersonic regime in an agar-gelatine gel. The entire experiment is completed in less than 10 milliseconds [106].

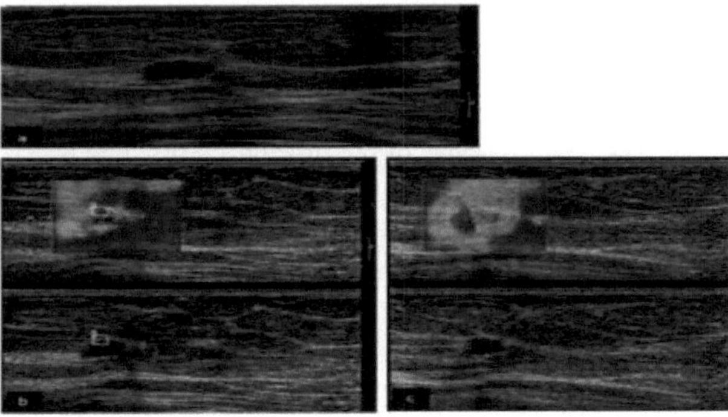

Fig. 11. shear wave elastography (a) lesion classified as BI-RADS 3 in B mode; **(b, c)** shear wave elastography. Elastographic mapping: the signal is heterogeneous hard in the periphery and the values are high. Max elasticity 180 kPa. The lesion is reclassified BI-RADS 4. Histology: invasive cancer type NST [107].

1.4.2.2.2. Acoustic Radiation Force Impulse (ARFI) technology

The "ARFI" or "Acoustic Radiation Force Imaging" mode is a method developed by K. Nightingale [108-110]. It also uses radiation pressure but employs a single focused ultrasound beam and does not analyse shear wave propagation, but the local displacement of the target secondane to the acoustic radiation force. The application of the radiation force slightly displaces the tissue at the focus according to Hooke's law. The transducer then switches to imaging mode and detects the displacement at the focus using ultrasound speckle interferometry.

The ultrasound speckle interferometry technique [111], previously used in static elastography, allows window-by-window correlation of the ultrasound signal to detect tissue displacement with sub-micrometre sensitivity. It is thus possible to follow the displacement and relaxation of the tissue as a function of the radiation force. In particular, the temporal properties of these relaxation curves make it possible to deduce information about elasticity and viscosity at the focal point only (fig.12) [112].

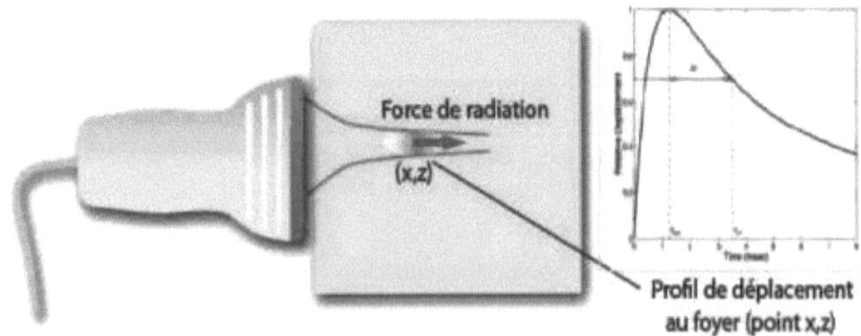

Fig. 12 Principle of ARFI elastography.

The radiation force is used to displace the tissue at the focus. Study of the displacement profile, in particular its maximum and relaxation time, provides information about the hardness of the medium. This displacement profile is estimated by axial cross-correlation of the speckle on the line corresponding to the focal point [72].

The ARFI technique also makes it possible to reconstruct a complete image by scanning the zone, but this has the disadvantage of increasing the acquisition time to form a complete image and depositing a lot of energy in the medium, which can cause considerable heating [113]. This module records the tangential displacement in the vicinity of the incident probe [114].

Gomme in Supersonic Shear Imaging, Nightingale et al. are also interested in the propagation of shear waves generated by radiation pressure and have proposed a new ARFI mode, allowing quantitative measurement of the Young's modulus [115].

ARFI elastography is quick and easy to use, in real time. Once the ARFI elastography mode has been selected, a short wave pulse (0.03-0.4 ms) of high acoustic power causes internal tissue excitation (displacement greater than 20 μ) in the zone of interest (ROI), which is captured by conventional acoustic probe focusing. The shots are successive and emitted at short intervals in order to follow the tissue displacements, the pulse-detection sequence is generated over the entire width of the ROI.

ARFI elastography combines a qualitative analysis (virtual touch imaging: VTI), which reproduces the hardness of an area of interest in grey scale or colour, and a quantitative analysis (virtual touch quantification: VTQ), which measures the mean speed of shear wave propagation in m/s by positioning a ROI of defined size. The velocity threshold for differentiating between benign and malignant masses varies between studies, ranging from 2 to more than 4 m/s [116-119]. In general, a velocity greater than 2 m/s is suggestive of a malignant lesion and vice versa (fig. 13).

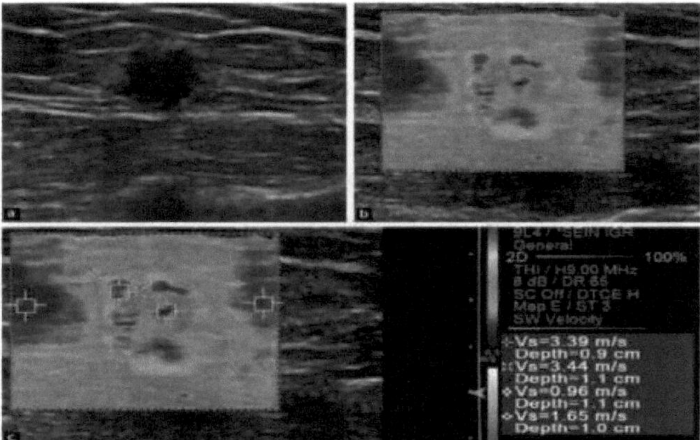

Fig. 13. ARFI mode elastography (Siemens®), (a) 6 mm lesion, microlobulated, suspicious; **(b)** slightly deformable lesion in colour ARFI mode, with predominant red and orange areas in and around the lesion. (c) the velocities measured in the lesion are very high (> 3 m/s), in favour of a malignant lesion. Histology:

NST infiltrating carcinoma, grade II [120].

1.4.3. Clinical applications

The main use of breast elastography is to improve the characterisation of benign and malignant lesions of the breast [86, 121]. Numerous studies have shown that the use of elastography parameters, in addition to ultrasound parameters, optimises the BI-RADS score [122, 123].

1.4.3.1. Benign breast lesions

The term "benign breast lesions" refers to a heterogeneous group of lesions that can present a wide range of symptoms.

The incidence of benign breast lesions increases during the second decade of life, with a peak in the fourth and fifth decades, unlike malignant pathology, whose incidence increases after the menopause, but at a slower rate [124].

Benign breast conditions can be diffuse lesions of the mammary gland or focal lesions.

In the first case, the increase in the epithelial and connective tissue component results in a vast ultrasound polymorphism, most often represented by microcysts and ductal dilatation. Certain pathologies, such as sclerosing adenosis, can generate images malignant lesions. Elastography adds important details to define the different tissue components and their elasticity, although this technique appears to be more useful in the study of focal lesions [125].

Benign focal lesions are usually round or oval in shape with a "wider than tall" appearance indicating an orientation that is parallel to the chest wall, usually with clear boundaries and regular contours. The echostructure may be hypoechoic (solid mass) or anechoic (cystic) and is often homogeneous. Vascularity is variable and depends on the histological nature of the mass.

In general, benign lesions are harder than normal breast tissue but softer than malignant tumours [126, 127]. Exceptions may occur and some benign lesions, such adenofibroma and cytosteatonecrosis, may be hard to palpate and may cause false positives on elastography [102].

Benign lesions are described by elastography as a lesion with a low colorimetric score (score 1 - 2), whereas the cut-off score for distinguishing between a benign and a malignant mass is 3 - 4 according to the Ueno-Itoh colorimetric classification [84].

On the subject elasticity and size ratios, various studies were carried out in 2010-2011. A meta-analysis by Sadigh [123] evaluated 12 articles from 3000 references. The elasticity ratio threshold varied from 0.5 to 4.5 in the different studies. The average sensitivity was 88%, with specificity of 83% for the elasticity ratio and 98% and 72% for the size ratio.

The experience obtained in the tissue quantification of breast lesions using the ARFf mode is extremely limited, represented by a few articles [116, 117, 128, 129].

In the most recent paper by Tozaki et al, on a series of 161 masses including 43 cancers, the threshold for differentiating benign and malignant lesions is 3.59 m/s [117], whereas it had previously been described as 3,065 m/s by Bai et al [119].
According to Tozaki, the average speed of shear wave propagation in 76.5% of malignant lesions is higher than in benign lesions (4.49 m/s vs 2.68 m/s).
In 23.5% of malignant lesions, measurement of shear wave velocity was not possible. The author concludes that the ARFf mode may be useful in diagnosing benign lesions. In practice, the benign/malignant differentiation threshold may vary from 2.20 m/s to 4.5 m/s depending on the studies that have evaluated this technique [116-118].
The results of a multicentre study carried out in 16 centres on almost 1800 patients are available and reported by Berg et al (BEI study) [130]. This study concerned the first 958 patients and 939 lesions, 289 of which were malignant. The most relevant and reproducible elastographic criteria are the shape of the lesion and the homogeneous or heterogeneous nature of the colour mapping and the maximum elasticity assessed on the colour scale or by measuring the maximum value (Emax) with a maximum elasticity threshold of 80 kPa in the hardest area of the lesion. Specificity was increased from 61.1% to 78.5% (77.4% for quantitative maximum elasticity Emax) without altering sensitivity. Malignancy rates for Bf-RADS 3 lesions were reduced to 1% (vs. 2.6%). The PPV of BI-RADS 4a lesions was more than doubled, reducing the number of unnecessary biopsies in this category (malignancy rate: 9.3%). The gain for the sub-group of oval and circumscribed masses (181 cases) is particularly interesting, with colour mapping enabling the identification of all cancers classified as BIRADS 3 (4 cases).
Complicated cysts were often associated with a multilayered appearance in elastographic colour mapping [90, 98]. This is probably an artefact in the colour distribution due to the scarcity of echoes, affecting the calculation elasticity and is often the cause of measurement errors [125].
On elastography, cysts can have variable elastographic appearances, often appearing as hard, poorly deformable lesions, generally represented in blue on colour mapping and with a high elasticity ratio, due to their low compressibility [86].
The elastographic properties of adenofibromas are controversial. Some studies report a substantial difference in fibrous components compared with the surrounding parenchyma [84], while other authors describe adenofibromas as difficult to assess by colour mapping because of their mammary gland-like elasticity [131, 132], with the range of elasticity ratio reported by most authors for this specific type of lesion being around 2.1 ± 0.8 [133]. Adenofibromas with a large fibrous component and low cell density may appear suspicious on colour mapping, but in all cases the elasticity ratio is lower than in malignant forms [84, 134].
Cytostatonecrosis occurs after physical trauma to the breast, whatever the nature

(surgical, biopsy, radiation, traumatic), is of variable ultrasound appearance, anechogenic cyst, homogeneous echogenic cyst, or with a fat-liquid level, can be very worrying in the presence of an attenuating irregular image. Progression towards sclerosis may give rise to controversial ultrasound images. Radial scarring or Aschoff's proliferative centre, for example, appears on imaging as an architectural distortion due to the fibrous reaction of the surrounding glandular tissue. It can be difficult to differentiate it from certain well-differentiated invasive cancers, the radiological expression of which is a very marked image of convergence.

Radial scarring is difficult to differentiate from malignant lesions because of the similar elastographic appearance in most . Cytosteonecrosis is reliably diagnosed on mammography, whereas radial scarring remains a diagnostic challenge that can only be verified by histological examination [135].

1.4.3.2. Malignant lesions of the breast

Breast cancer usually presents as a focal lesion with malignant features such as an irregular mass, irregular or even spiculated contours, posterior acoustic attenuation, an echogenic peripheral halo with a desmoplastic reaction around the lesion, calcifications and significant vascularisation on Doppler.

The malignant lesion may also have non-specific features such as architectural distortion and diffuse redema of the gland [136]. The diffuse form is typical of carcinomas with inflammatory features, in which there is thickening of the cutaneous yolk, abnormal echogenicity of the breast and dilation of the cutaneous and subcutaneous lymphatic vessels in the form of anechogenic bands.

Tumour hardness is a characteristic of the extracellular matrix (abnormally firm stroma), modulated by collagen and activated fibroblasts, and is known as desmoplastic transformation [137]. Malignant lesions are less deformable than healthy breast tissue and have a more complex modulus of elasticity [103], in agreement with the results of the study by Krouskop et al [73].

Some breast cancers may appear deformable, with a pseudobenign appearance on elastography, such as medullary, mucinous and papillary tumours, certain non-specific necrotic infiltrating carcinomas and lesions smaller than 5 mm because they have little reaction stroma [102, 138]. Some of these lesions may even appear as cysts on elastography (mucinous cancers) [131, 134, 139].

Giuseppetti et al [139] in their study (91 nodules, 27 benign, 64 malignant) noted that histological type and lesion size influence the degree of elasticity. Ductal forms may have different patterns of elasticity depending on their fibrohyaline component and the stage of the tumour (a small ductal tumour tends to have a smaller fibrous component). Lobular forms have particular histopathological features, such as low cellularity, low fibrohyaline component and moderate desmoplastic reaction, particularly in small lesions. This study demonstrated that static elastography has a sensitivity and specificity of 79% and 89% respectively in the diagnosis of benign versus malignant masses. Elastography is mainly used for suspicious lesions, classified as BI - RADS 3 and 4, but management does not change in the case of BI-RADS 1, 2 and 5 lesions [85, 86].

Zhi et al [87] compared mammography, ultrasound and static elastography in the evaluation of masses in dense breasts. The study included 296 lesions (209 benign, 87 malignant). Elastography achieved the highest specificity (95.7%) and the lowest false positive rate (4.3%) compared with the other methods. Most false negatives occur in non-specific infiltrating carcinomas with a large central area of necrosis. The combination of ultrasound and static elastography improved sensitivity (89.7%), specificity (95.7%), false negative rate (9.2%) and PPV (89.7%).

Semi-quantitative examination using static elastography shows that malignant lesions have a high elasticity ratio (between 2 [140] and 3.52 [141]) and a high size ratio, greater than 1 [142].

Barr et al [142] presented the results of a multicentre study including 222 malignant and atypical lesions and 431 benign lesions. A size ratio greater than 1 was found in 219 malignant lesions out of 222, and a size ratio less than 1 was found in 361 benign lesions out of 431, giving a sensitivity of 98.6% and a specificity of 87.4%. Lesion size on elastography appeared to correlate better with histological size.

Using the ARFI technique, malignant masses have higher values than benign lesions, as demonstrated in the study by Bai et al [119] with velocity values between 2.25 ± 0.59 m/s for benign lesions and around 5.96 ± 2.96 m/s for malignant lesions.

Tozaki et al [117] studied a series of 161 masses including 43 cancers, using a threshold of 3.6 m/s to differentiate between benign and malignant lesions to obtain a sensitivity of 91% with a specificity of 80.6%.

Examination of malignant lesions using shear waves, in the study by Athanasiou et al [102], gave a mean elasticity value of 146.6 kPa

± 40.05 ($\rho < 0.001$), while benign masses had an elasticity value of 45.3 kPa ±41.1 ($p < 0.001$). Complex cysts were differentiated from solid lesions by an elasticity value of 0 kPa. Shear wave elastography showed higher specificity than ultrasound (96% vs 63%), while sensitivity was similar for both methods (95% and 96%).

1.4.3.3. Limits

Breast elastography has a number of limitations, mainly related to the density of glandular tissue and breast mass, but also to the elastographic technique.

The high density of breast tissue can lead to false-negative breast lesions [143]. Elastography evaluates the elasticity and deformability of lesions in comparison with the surrounding tissue, and this can sometimes be a source of misinterpretation.

Appropriate compression is also an important factor that can influence the elasticity

factor, particularly in static elastography [144]. The general recommendation is that the transducer should be in very light contact with the skin at the start of the examination because compression and elasticity are no longer proportional beyond a certain degree of compression [145-147].
Assessment should be carried out with greater precision for superficial lesions than for deep lesions, given the size of the breasts [143,145], while a lesion close to the nipple makes it difficult to obtain optimum image quality [128].
More studies are needed to investigate these issues further, as no studies have yet been carried out that take into account the depth of the lesion, the size of the lesion, and whether or not it is palpable.
Finally, only a few studies describe the correlation between histological features and elastography results, so the diagnosis and clinical performance of elastography in different types of lesions are not yet fully known.

2. Issues

Breast ultrasound is a highly sensitive imaging technique, with sensitivity of over 90%, but specificity is low to moderate and varies according to the series, without taking into account technical advances such high-frequency probes, harmonic and composite modes and colour Doppler, combined with semiological analysis according to the ACR BI-RADS lexicon [10].
The American College of Radiology Imaging Network (ACRIN) has evaluated the added value of ultrasound in mammographic screening, by comparing mammography alone with the combination of mammography and ultrasound in high-risk patients with dense breasts [147]. The sensitivity of screening was increased by 27% with the addition of ultrasound, but with a loss of specificity of 6.12% [148].
On the other hand, biopsy rates have increased from 3.2% to 5.2% and the positive predictive value of biopsy for these lesions found by ultrasound is low estimated at 8.9% compared with 22.6% for those found by mammography. In addition, these false-positive ultrasound findings are frequently responsible for unnecessary surveillance, of approximately 8.6% of lesions versus 2.2% of lesions detected by mammography [149].
Ultrasound has certain limitations, both in terms of detecting and characterising lesions:

- differentiation between solid and liquid masses ;
- identification of cyst contents ;
- estimating the size of lesions ;
- detection and characterisation of isoechoic fat lesions and deep lesions;
- Visualisation of cancers that develop by diffuse extension without a mass syndrome, such as infiltrating lobular cancers and endocanal cancers;
- non-discriminatory vascularisation.

Furthermore, the reproducibility of the final BI-RADS is low, estimated overall at 0.28; it is better for lesions classified as BI-RADS 5, at 0.56, 0.32 for BI-RADS 3 categories and very low for lesions classified as BIRADS 4a and 4b, estimated at 0.14 and 0.16 respectively [150].

In this context, elastography methods have been developed which assess the hardness (or elasticity) of tissues or their relative displacements to provide an image of elasticity or deformation.

In order to situate ultrasound elastography in the context of other imaging studies in the management of breast lesions, we have set ourselves the goal of meeting the objectives of this study:

Does elastography improve the radiologist's ability to characterise breast lesions?

Can it reduce the number of biopsies of benign breast lesions?

Does it improve the management of certain lesions by avoiding unnecessary follow-up?

CHAPTER 2

Our study

Materials and methods

1. Objectives

The main objective of our study is:

To determine the diagnostic performance of ultrasound elastography in characterising benign and malignant breast lesions.

The secondary objectives of our study are:

- Analyse the elastographic characteristics of breast lesions according to :
- their palpable nature;
- their visibility in mammography;
- their size;
- their histological type;
- their infiltrating nature;
- the Scarff-Bloom and Richardson (SBR) histo-pronostic grade and the tumour's potential to evolve;
- To assess the influence of lesion size and depth on the diagnostic performance of elastography.

2. Materials and methods

This is a prospective study, 330 patients, carried out in the Medical Imaging Department of the Pierre and Marie Curie Centre (CPMC), fromJanuary 2016 toJanuary 2018.

2.1. Recruitment

Patients recruited from the imaging department of the Centre Pierre et Marie Curie with an ultrasound mass classified as 3, 4 or 5 according to the ACR ultrasound BIRADS classification [10], discovered during screening or at the time of a clinical abnormality.

Data were collected on a standardised data sheet and stored in a computer database. These forms included the patient's identity, age, sex, interview data, clinical examination data and the results of radiological investigations as well as those of histological sampling (appendix 2).

2.1.1. Inclusion criteria

Patients with a BI-RADS 3, 4 or 5 ultrasound mass with an elastographic study and a histological sample were included in this study.

2.1.2. Non-inclusion criteria

Patients with :

- An inconclusive biopsy result,
- a lesion classed 2 according to the ACR BI-RADS ultrasound classification [10],
- an extra-mammary mass (mastectomy wall and lymph node),
- underwent surgery, radiotherapy or neoadjuvant chemotherapy for contralateral or neighbouring lesions.

2.2. Sample size

- This involves calculating the number of subjects required (N) to estimate a proportion (sensitivity and specificity).

Sensitivity (Se) is the ratio $Se = \frac{\text{vrais positifs (VP)}}{\text{vrais positifs (VP)} + \text{faux négatifs(FN)}}$

Knowing also that the prevalence

(PR) : $PR = \frac{VP+FN}{N}$ et $VP + FN = \frac{\varepsilon^2 \times Se \times (1-Se)}{i^2}$

- The number of subjects required was calculated using the following formula:

$$N = \frac{\varepsilon^2 \times Se \times (1-Se)}{i^2} \Big/ PR = \frac{\varepsilon^2 \times Se \times (1-Se)}{i^2 \times PR}$$

- ε = 1.96 for a risk a = 0.05 - Sensitivity ranged from 77.6 to 87% [64, 76,110], with an average of 85%.

- i (precision): 0.075

- According to the CPMC pathology , the number of biopsies performed between 2012 and 2014 was 1644 (N), of which 480 were malignant (*NA*).

- Prevalence was calculated using the following formula:

$$PR = \frac{NA}{N} = \frac{480}{1644} = 0{,}29 \cong 0{,}3$$

The number of subjects required :

$$N = \frac{\varepsilon^2 \times Se \times (1-Se)}{i^2 \times PR} = \frac{1{,}96^2 \times 0{,}85 \times (1-0{,}85)}{0{,}075^2 \times 0{,}3} = 290{,}25$$

$\cong$ **300 subjects required**

2.3. Diagnostic means

2.3.1. Clinical examination

All patients were examined. The examination included questioning, inspection and palpation of both breasts, the axillary extensions and the supraclavicular hollows. Data the clinical examination were recorded on an individual form for each patient (appendix 2-1).

2.3.2. Mammography

The examinations were carried out using a HOLOGIC SELENIA digital mammography unit, commissioned in 2011.

Mammography was carried out as part of screening (women aged 40 and over) or in patients with a mass highly suspicious of malignancy on clinical examination or ultrasound.

All our patients underwent the same examination protocol. This protocol consisted of performing mammography bilaterally. It included two fundamental views, frontal and oblique. The additional views, i.e. profile, localised images and enlargements, were carried out on a case-by-case basis.

The images were analysed on a Soft Copy workstation.

For patients who have had a mammogram, we need to identify whether the mass is visible, whether there are microcalcifications and look any associated signs.
The interpretation of the mammographic images was based on the ACR BI-RADS mammographic classification [10]. Mammography data were collected on an individual form for each patient (appendix 2-2).
For all patients, mammographic images printed on Agfa film and burnt onto a CD-Rom for archiving.

2.3.3. Ultrasound

The examinations were carried out using a HITACHI "HI-VISION Avius" ultrasound machine, commissioned in January 2016. The machine is equipped two linear probes with multi-frequency transducers from 10 to 14 MHz.

2.3.3.1. Examination technique

All our patients underwent the same examination protocol. This protocol consisted of carrying out an ultrasound examination of the breasts bilaterally and comparatively. It included exploration of both breasts, the sub-mammary folds, the axillary hollows and the inter-mammary space.
The analysis of the breast lesion was devoted firstly to a morphological study in B mode and secondly to the analysis of vascularisation in colour Doppler mode.
The patient lay supine and was then optimally positioned to analyse the mass. The transducer was applied perpendicular to the chest wall, opposite the mass to be analysed. Two different frequency probes were used: the high-frequency linear strip probe (614 Mhz) was often used because of its better resolution, while the 2nd low-frequency linear probe (5-10 Mhz) had better penetration and was only used in large breasts with deep lesions. The usual processing of the ultrasound signal (gain, filter, frequency, focus and harmonic imaging) required for optimum image interpretation was applied according to the depth of the lesion.
Colour Doppler analysis was performed using standardised parameters (repetition frequency [low ERP between 700 and 1000 Hz], lowest possible wall filter [50-100 Hz], maximum Doppler gain [85-90%] and adaptation of the size of the Doppler box, without angulation).

2.3.3.2. Parameters analysed

Each mass was classified according to the ACR BI-RADS ultrasound classification [10], taking into account shape, orientation, contours, interface, echostructure, posterior acoustic signs and any calcifications (appendix 1).
The vascularisation of the mass was interpreted according to the groups described by Raza and Baum [45], distinguishing between no vascular flow, peripheral or centric flow and peripheral and central vascularisation.
The largest measurement in millimetres (mm) was chosen after measuring the mass in the three axes of space.
On ultrasound, other parameters were also analysed: the distance of the mass from the nipple, the distance between the anterior surface of the mass and the skin, and

the thickness of the breast from the upper edge of the pectoral muscle to the skin.

2.3.3.3. Data collection

Ultrasound data were collected on a form for each mass (appendix 2-3). The ultrasound images were reproduced on paper and on an external hard disk for storage.

2.3.4. Elastography

The elastographic examination was performed during the ultrasound analysis of the lesions using the elastography function of the ultrasound . Once the masses had been detected in B mode, elastography was performed for each lesion.

2.3.4.1. Examination technique

The transducer was applied perpendicular to the chest wall, opposite the mass to be analysed. The focusing of the image applied to the ultrasound image is not used with elastography. The pressure movement perpendicular to the chest wall, keeping the mass at the centre of the analysis window, must be repeated until a constant colour signal is obtained for at least 10 seconds. This video sequence is recorded and several sequences are sometimes necessary for optimal analysis of the mass. Movement depends on the depth of the mass, but the maximum depression is 1 to 2 mm. The average examination time per mass is 1 minute. As this is a dynamic examination, at least two acquisition cycles with identical results guarantee a correct technique. A digital scale checks the quality of movement with the transducer in real time, enabling immediate correction to achieve a technically optimal examination.

The colour analysis window, unlike the Doppler, must be very wide to analyse the behaviour of the mass and adjacent tissue. Two windows appear on the screen: the elastographic image on the left and the corresponding B mode ultrasound image on the right.

2.3.4.2. Parameters analysed

Various qualitative and quantitative parameters were analysed on the elastographic image.

2.3.4.2.1. Study of qualitative parameters

- Homogeneity of mapping: homogeneous, not very homogeneous, heterogeneous.
- Maximum colour.
- Location the hardest area: intra, peri, intra and peri lesion.
- Intra-lesion echo pressure: echo presence / echo void.

- Classify the colour mapping according to the classification proposed by Itoh in 5 categories [84] (fig. 5), completely soft (scores 1,2), rather soft (score 3), rather hard (score 4) and hard inside and at the periphery of the mass (score 5).

o Score 1: mass is green, like the surrounding tissue;

- Score 2: three colours not arranged in layers (mosaic of green, blue, red);
- Score 3: the mass is blue and the peripheral part is green;
- Score 4: the entire mass is blue;
- Score 5: the entire mass and the peripheral zone are blue.

2.3.4.2.2. Study of quantitative parameters

- Elasticity ratio

For the semi-quantitative assessment of mass elasticity, we manually positioned regions of interest (ROIs) on the same colour map. Two quantitative parameters were obtained:

Fat-Lesion **Ratio** FLR), with the first ROI plotted on the colour map in the lesion (L) and the second ROI in the subcutaneous fat (F). The F to L ratio (FLR= F / L) is expressed as a standard deviation (fig. 14 a).

Glande-Lesion **Ratio (**GLR), the first ROI plotted on the colour map in the lesion (L) and the second ROI in the glandular tissue (G). The G to L ratio (GLR= G / L), expressed as standard deviation (fig. 14b).

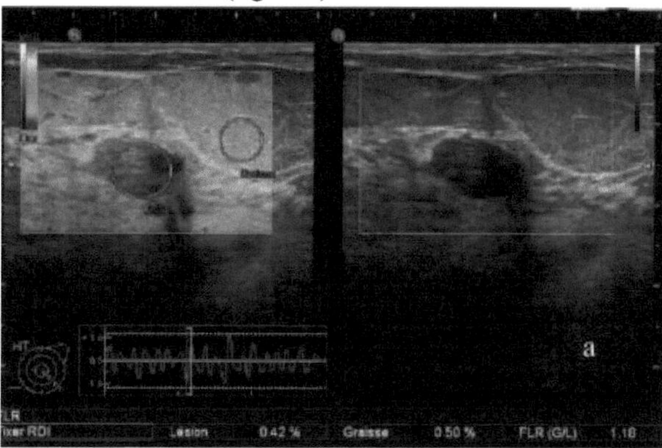

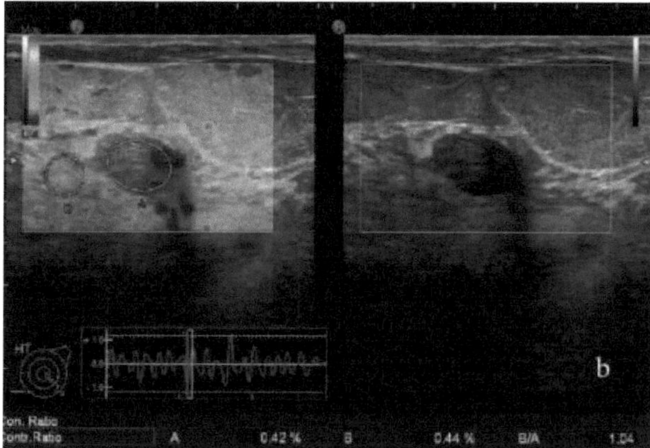

Fig. 14. elasticity ratio. (a) Fat-to-lesion ratio = FLR, the first ROI plotted on the colour map in

the lesion (L) and the second ROI in the subcutaneous fat (F). The F to L ratio (FLR= F / L), in this example calculated at 1.18. (b) *Glande-Lesion* Ratio (= GLR), The first ROI plotted on the colour map in the lesion (L) and the second ROI in the glandular tissue (G). The G to L ratio (GLR= G / L), calculated at 1.04. Histology: fibroadenoma.

Size ratio

The size ratio is the ratio of the longest axis of the lesion measured on the elastographic image and the longest axis of the corresponding image measured on B-mode ultrasound (fig. 15).

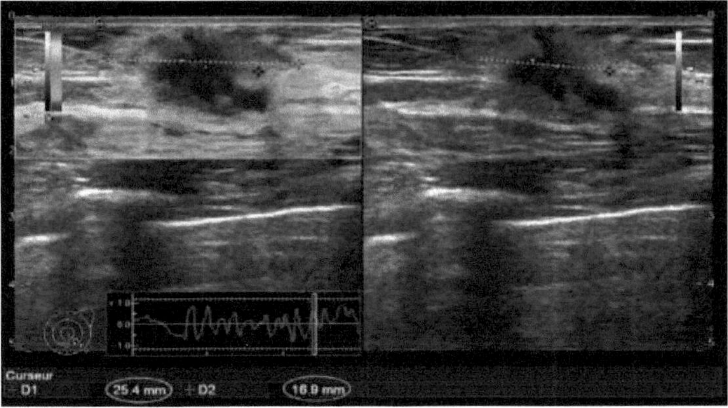

Fig. 15 Size ratio. The ratio of the longest axis of the lesion measured on the elastographic image and the longest axis of the corresponding image measured on B-mode ultrasound. The size ratio in this example is calculated as 1.50. Histology: Invasive carcinomaNST.

2.3.4.3. Combination of B mode ultrasound and elastographic parameters

Based on the combination of B-mode ultrasound and elastographic parameters, we reclassified masses by downgrading by one BI-RADS category lesions that had elasticity score, elasticity ratio and size values below the threshold values.

2.3.4.4. Data collection

Elastographic data was collected on a form for each mass (appendix 2-4). The elastographic images reproduced on paper and on an external hard disk for storage.

2.3.5. Histological study

In order to carry out an anatomopathological analysis of the lesions, a percutaneous biopsy under ultrasound control is necessary, subject to a correct haemostasis assessment. An informed consent form was submitted to the patient, collecting their personal data and informing them of the procedure and the risks involved (appendix 3). We used a Bard® automatic sampling system with 14 gauge needles for the 352 microbiopsies, while 23 macrobiopsies were carried out using the Vacora® system with a 10 gauge needle.

The analysis was carried out by a single pathologist from the Centre Pierre et Marie

Curie.

The lesions were divided into two groups, benign and malignant, using the histological results as the reference examination.

Benign masses were classified according to their histological type. Fibroepithelial lesions were classified into three groups according to their stremal cellularity: low or moderate cellularity for fibroadenomas and highly cellular stroma for phyllodes tumours [151].

Histological analysis in the case of malignant tumours included the following elements, obtained as part of the usual routine histological analysis: histological type, SBR tumour grade, hormone receptors (restrogens, progesterone), HER2 status and Ki 67 proliferation index.

Of the 72 patients with malignant lesions, only 37 operative reports (lumpectomy or mastectomy) were retrieved from the pathology department. The remaining 35 either underwent neoadjuvant treatment or underwent surgery outside our establishment.

Analysis of the amount of fibrosis, the presence or absence of vascular emboli, necrosis or mucin, and identification of the long axis of the mass were carried out on the surgical specimen.

These histological parameters were then correlated with the elasticity parameters obtained by elastographic analysis.

Data from percutaneous samples and surgical specimens were collected on individual forms for each patient (appendices 2-5 and 2-6) and recorded on computer software.

2.3.6. Statistical analysis

Statistical analyses carried out using SPSS 23 software.

- Descriptive statistics

Quantitative variables are represented by means and standard deviations, qualitative variables by number of cases and percentage.

- The tests used

- The Student's t-test is used to compare two means or the ANOVA test to compare several means.
- The $\chi 2$ test or Fisher's exact test, to compare percentages.
- The Spearman correlation test (rho) is used to estimate the relationship between a qualitative ordinal variable and a quantitative variable.
- The Pearson correlation test (r) is used to estimate the relationship between two quantitative variables.

- Analysis of diagnostic performance

- Performance is assessed using an ROC curve (the ROC curve is the plot of sensitivity values as a function of 1-specificity for the different thresholds in the test).

- The choice of threshold values was obtained using the Youden index (sensitivity + specificity -1) [152].
- The area under the curve (AUC), sensitivity, specificity, positive predictive value (PPV), negative predictive value (NPV) and accuracy are calculated for each examination (ultrasound mode B, elasticity score, elasticity ratio and size ratio) (appendix 4).
- The McNemar test and the $\chi2$ test are used to compare the AUC, sensitivity, specificity, accuracy, PPV and NPV of B-mode ultrasound alone to different elastographic parameters and to B-mode ultrasound and elastography combinations.

For all tests, a p-value of less than 0.05 is taken as the significance threshold.

Results

Our prospective study was conducted fromJanuary 2016 toJanuary 2018 over a 24-month period. It included a total of 330 patients, 72 of whom had malignant breast masses (malignant group) and 258 patients with benign breast masses (benign group).

Patients were recruited and explored in the Medical Imaging Department of the Pierre and Marie Curie Centre.

1. Description of the study population

1.1. Gender

The study population comprised 328 female patients (99.39%) and two male patients (0.61%), with a clear female predominance.

258 (100%) patients, all female, had benign masses and 72 patients, including two males, had malignant masses (Table 1).

Table 1. Distribution of benign and malignant groups according to sex.			
Patient	**Benin n = 258**	**Malignant n = 72**	**P**
Gender			0,07
Woman	258 (100 %)	70 (97 %)	
Men	0	2 (3 %)	

1.2. Age

The mean age of the patients was 43.82 years, with a standard deviation of 13.97 years, and extremes of 16-92 years.

Patients with benign masses were younger than those with malignant masses (mean age 41.80 versus 55.47 respectively;< *0.0001*) (Table 2).

Table 2. Average age of the benign and malignant groups.			
Patient	**Benign n = 258**	**Malignant n = 72**	***P***
Age (years)			**< 0,001**
Mean + Standard deviation	41,80 ±12,30	55,47 + 13,04	
Min-max	16-78	31-92	

The breakdown of the population by 10-year age group shows that the 45-55 age group accounts for 30.30% of the population studied.

The peak age range was identical for subjects in both the benign and malignant groups *(p^_l)* (fig. 16).

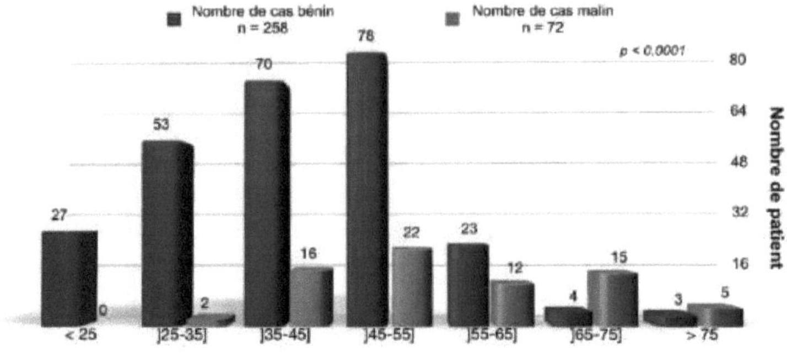

Fig. 16. Distribution of cases according to age group in the benign and malignant groups.

1.3. Body mass index (BMI)

The BMI of the population studied was between 15.6 and 46.

The distribution of the population according to BMI showed that 61.21% of patients were overweight (overweight and obese).

Among patients with malignant tumours, 77.78% were overweight, compared with 56.58% in the group with benign tumours (*p = 0.001*) (table 3).

Table 3. BMI distribution of benign and malignant groups.

Patient	**Benin η = 258**	**Malignant η = 72**	***P***
BMI			***0,002***
Leanness < 18.5	16 (6,20 %)	0	
Normal [18.5-25[	96 (37,21 %)	16 (22,22 %)	
Overweight [25-30[	98 (37,98 %)	32 (44,44 %)	
Obesity > 30	48(18,60%)	24 (33,33 %)	

1.4. Genital activity

217 (65.76%) patients were genitally active, with an average age of 37.55 years and a standard deviation of 9.20 years.

12 patients were pre-menopausal, with an average age of 49.75 years and a standard deviation of 2.50 years.

99 patients were postmenopausal, with a mean age of 59.42 years and a standard deviation of 9.31 years.

The majority (55.72%) of patients a malignant mass were menopausal (52.86%) or pre-menopausal (2.86%), while 72.09% of patients with a benign mass were genitally active (p = 0.004) (Table 4).

Table 4. Distribution according to genital activity of the benign and malignant groups.

Pariente	**Benin n = 258**	**Malignant n = 70**	***P***

Genital activity			0,00007
Non-menopausal	186 (72,09 %)	31 (44,29 %)	
Pre-menopausal	10 (3,88 %)	2 (2,86 %)	
Menopausal	62 (24,03 %)	37 (52,86 %)	

1.5. Menarchy

Menarcheal age in the study population ranged from 9 to 19 years, with an average of 13.42 + 1.58 years.

Early menarche less than or equal to 11 years of age was found in 7.75% of benign cases versus 8.57% of malignant cases, with no significant difference *(p = 0.8).*

Table 5 shows the age distribution of patients with benign and malignant masses.

Table 5. Age of benign and malignant menarche.

Pariente	Benin n = 258	Malignant n = 70	P
Age of menarchy (years)			0,17
<11	20 (7,75%)	6 (8,57%)	
12	67 (25,97%)	13 (18,57%)	
13	61 (23,64%)	17 (24,29%)	
14	56(21,71%)	17 (24,29%)	
15	24 (9,30%)	11 (15,71%)	
16	19 (7,36%)	2 (2,86%)	
> 17	11 (4,26%)	4(5,71%)	

1.6. Menopause

For the 99 menopausal patients (30.18%), the age at menopause was between 35 and 60 years, with an average of 48.31+4.71 years.

The mean age at menopause for patients with benign masses and for patients with malignant masses was 47.85 + 4.42 years (35-57 years) and 49.08 + 5.13 years (36-60 years) respectively *(ρ = 0.21).*

Late menopause occurring after the age of 55 was noted in 5 (8.06%) parients in the benign group and in 6 (16.22%) parients in the malignant group, with no significant difference *(p = 0.32)* (table 6).

Table 6. Distribution of benign and malignant groups according to age at menopause.

Patient	Benin n = 62	Malin n = 37	P
Age at menopause (years)			0,33
[35-40[	2 (3,23%)	2(5,41%)	
[40-45 [	7(11,29%)	3 (8,11%)	
[45-50[	29 (46,77%)	13 (35,14%)	
[50-55[	19 (30,65%)	13 (35,14%)	
[55-60]	5 (8,06%)	6 (16,22%)	

1.7. Pregnancy

The number of pregnancies in the study population ranged from 0 to 12, with an average of 1.99 ±2.41.

The average number of pregnancies for women with malignant tumours was higher than for women with benign lesions (2.93 + 2.83 versus 1.88 ± 2.3, p = *0.0026).*

The distribution of the population according to the number of pregnancies shows a peak for women with 3 pregnancies in the benign and malignant groups combined (fig. 17).

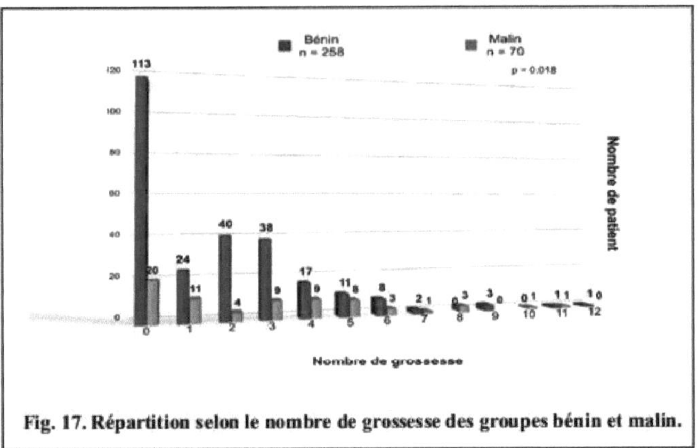

Fig. 17. Répartition selon le nombre de grossesse des groupes bénin et malin.

Fig. 17: Distribution of benign and malignant groups according to the number of pregnancies.

1.8. Parity

The number of parities in the population studied ranged from 0 to 12, with an average of 1.86 + 2.25.

The average number of parities for males with a malignant tumour was higher than for females with a benign lesion (2.74 + 2.68 versus 1.76 ± 2.13, p = *0.0025).*

The distribution of the population according to the number of parities in patients with benign and malignant masses is shown in Figure 18.

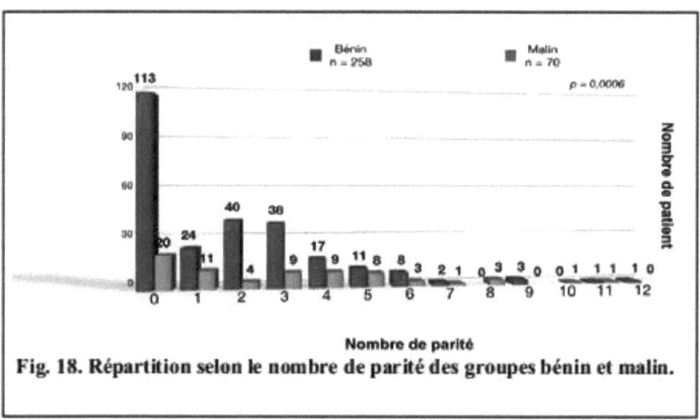

Fig. 18. Répartition selon le nombre de parité des groupes bénin et malin.

Fig. 18. Distribution of benign and malignant groups by number of parities

1.9. Age of first pregnancy

The average age at first pregnancy of the parents was 24.89 + 5.81 years (1445 years).

The mean age at first pregnancy for women with benign and malignant masses was 25.07 +5.34 years (14-42 years) and 23.94 +7.17 years (14-45 years) respectively *(p = 0.1)*.

Late age at first pregnancy (30 years and over) was found in 31 (21.22%) parientes in the benign group and in 11 (22%) parientes in the malignant group (p = 0.68) (table 7).

Table 7. Distribution according to age at first pregnancy of the benign and malignant groups.

Patient	**Benin n = 146**	**Malignant n = 50**	***P***
Age at first pregnancy (years)			0,05
<20	16 (10,96 %)	14 (28,00 %)	
[20-25 [	54 (36,99 %)	15 (30,00 %)	
[25-30[	45 (30,82 %)	10 (20,00 %)	
[30-35[	21 (14,38 %)	7 (14,00 %)	
[35-40[	9(6,16%)	2 (4,00 %)	
>40	1 (0,68 %)	2 (4,00 %)	

1.10. Breastfeeding

178 subjects had breastfed and 150 had not, i.e. 45.73% (Table 8).

The distribution of the population according to breastfeeding status showed that 54.27% had breastfed, including 24.71% with malignant tumours and 75.29% with benign tumours *(p < 0.0001)*.

The duration of breastfeeding in the population studied ranged from 0 to 168 months, with an average of 42.22 + 40.73 months.

The average duration of breastfeeding in parity with benign and malignant masses was 40.99 + 39.20 months (0-168 months) and 52.57 + 47.01 months (3-168 months) respectively *(p = 0.17)*.

Table 8. Distribution of benign and malignant groups according to breastfeeding.			
Patient	**Benin n = 258**	**Malignant n = 70**	***P***
Breastfeeding			0,10
Breastfeeding	134 (51,94%)	44 (63 %)	
Not breastfeeding	124 (48,06 %)	26 (37 %)	

1.11. Oral contraception

32.01% of the population studied had taken oral contraception.
Use of oral contraception was 34% in patients with malignant tumours and 31.40% in patients with benign tumours (φ- *0.65)* (table 9).

Table 9. Distribution of benign and malignant groups according to use of oral contraception.			
Patient	**Benin n = 258**	**Malignant n = 70**	***P***
Contraception			0,65
Yes	81 (31,40%)	24 (34 %)	
No	177 (68,60 %)	46 (66 %)	

The duration of oral contraceptive use in the study population ranged from 0 to 24 years, with an average of 5.93 + 5.27 years.
The mean duration of oral contraceptive use by patients with benign and malignant masses was 5.69 ±5.19 years (0-24 years) and 7.79 + 5.62 years (1-20 years) respectively *(p = 0.1)*.

1.12. Hormonal treatment

Seven patients had taken hormonal treatment to ovulation, 4 patients had a benign mass and 3 patients had a malignant mass *(p = 0.35)*.
The mean duration of hormone treatment for patients with benign and malignant masses was 2.25 + 1.89 years (1-5 years) and 0.33 + 0.58 years (0-1 years) respectively *(p = 0.06)*.

1.13. History

1.13.1. Personal history

No patient in the study population had a history of surgery, radiotherapy or neoadjuvant chemotherapy for a contralateral or neighbouring breast lesion, which are exclusion criteria in our study.

1.13.2. Family history

67 patients had a family history of breast or ovarian cancer, i.e.
20.30% of the population studied (table 10).

Table 10. Distribution of benign and malignant groups according to family history of breast cancer.			
Patient	**Benin η = 258**	**Malignant η = 72**	*P*
Family history			0,76
Breast cancer	51 (19,77%)	13 (18 %)	
Ovarian cancer	2 (0,78 %)	i (i %)	
CLEAR	205 (79,46 %)	58(81 %)	

64 patients had a family history of breast cancer, including 51 patients with a benign breast lesion and 13 patients with a malignant breast lesion *(p = 0.75).*
Their mean ages at diagnosis in the benign and malignant groups were 49.29 + 12.99 years (20-90 years) and 47.15 + 15.87 years (19-79 years) respectively *(p = 0.06).*
Of the 64 patients with a family history of breast cancer, 46 patients had a first-degree relative and 18 patients had a second-degree relative.
The distribution of benign and malignant groups according to family history of breast cancer is shown in table 11.

Table 11. Distribution according to degree of relatedness of family history of breast cancer in the benign and malignant groups.			
Patient	**Benin n = 51**	**Malignant n = 13**	*P*
Degree of family history of breast cancer			0,91
First degree (mother, sister or son-in-law)	36 (70,59 %)	10 (77 %)	
Second degree (grandmother, aunt, niece)	15 (29,41 %)	3 (23 %)	

Three patients had a family history of ovarian cancer, including two patients with a benign breast lesion and one with a malignant breast lesion *(p = 0.82).*

2. Clinical characteristics

2.1. Reason for consultation

The majority of patients with benign masses consulted for screening (115 out of 258 or 44.57% of benign patients vs 13 out of 72 or 18.06% of malignant patients, *p = 0.00004*), unlike patients with malignant lesions who often consulted for a palpable mass (52 out of 72 (72.22%) of malignant patients vs 72 out of 258 (27.91%) of benign patients, *p = 0.0001*) (see Table 12).

Table 12. Breakdown of benign and malignant groups by reason for consultation.			
Patient	**Benin n = 258**	**Malignant n = 72**	***P***
Reason for consultation			**< 0,0001**
Screening	115 (44,57 %)	13 (18,06%)	
Mastodynia	69 (26,74 %)	4 (5,56 %)	
Mass	72 (27,91 %)	52 (72,22 %)	

Other	2 (0,78 %)	3 (4,17%)	

2.2. Clinical examination

2.2.1. Inspection

2.2.1.1. Breast contours

93% of the population studied had no change in breast contour, 97.67% of patients a benign lesion versus 76.39% of patients a malignant lesion *(p < 0.0001).*

23 patients changes in breast contour, such as curvature (5 out of 72 malignant patients vs. 4 out of 258 benign patients, *p = 0.038*) and retraction (12 out of 72 malignant patients vs. 2 out of 258 benign patients, *p < 0.0001*) (table 13).

Table 13. Distribution by breast contour of the benign and malignant groups.			
Patient	**Benin η = 258**	**Malignant η = 72**	***P***
Breast contour			**0,0001**
Normal	252 (97,67 %)	55 (76,39 %)	
Youure	4(1,55%)	5 (6,94 %)	
Flat	0	0	
Shrinkage	2 (0,78 %)	12(16,67%)	

2.2.1.2. Skin changes

97.9% of the population studied had no skin changes, 98.84% of patients with a benign lesion versus 94.44% of patients with a malignant lesion *(p = 0.022).*

Nine patients showed skin changes, of the reddening type (1 out of 72 malignant patients vs. 1 out of 258 benign patients, *p = 0.91*) and of the thickening type (3 out of 72 malignant patients vs. 2 out of 258 benign patients,^ = *0.12*) (table 14).

Table 14. Distribution of benign and malignant groups according to skin changes.			
Patient	**Benin n = 258**	**Malignant n = 72**	*P*
Skin changes			*0,08*
Absence	255 (98,84 %)	68 (94,44 %)	
Redness	1 (0,39 %)	1 (1,39%)	
Skin thickening	2 (0,78 %)	3 (4,17 %)	
Orange peel skin	0	0	

2.2.1.3. Changes to the nipple

97.3% of the population studied had no nipple changes, 99.61% of patients with benign lesions versus 88.89% of patients malignant lesions *(p < 0.0001).*

Nine patients skin changes, umbilication type (3 out of 72 malignant patients vs 1 out of 258 benign patients, *p = 0.047*) and retraction type (5 out of 72 malignant patients) (table 15).

Table 15. Distribution according to nipple changes of the benign and malignant groups.			
Patient	**Benin η = 258**	**Malignant η = 72**	***P***
Changes to the nipple			**0,0001**
Absence	257 (99,61 %)	64 (88,89 %)	
Umbilical	1 (0,39 %)	3 (4,17 %)	
Shrinkage	0	5 (6,94 %)	
Eczematiform erosion	0	0	

2.2.2. Palpation

62.9% of the population studied had no palpable lesion, and 37.1% of lesions were palpable in the form of a mass or placard (table 16).

No discharge or skin redema was noted on clinical examination.

Table 16. Distribution of benign and malignant masses according to palpation findings.			
Mass	**Benign n = 298**	**Malignant n = 77**	***P***
Palpation			**< 0,0001**
No lesions	217 (72,82 %)	19 (24,68 %)	
Cupboard	2 (0,67 %)	0	
Mass	79 (26,51 %)	58 (75,32 %)	
Flow	0	0	
cutaneous ffidema	0	0	

2.2.2.1. Mass

36.5% of the masses in our study were palpable (table 17).

Malignant masses were more often palpable (58/77) than benign masses (79/298*) (p < 0.0001).*

Table 17. Distribution of benign and malignant masses according to palpation.			
Mass	**Benign η = 298**	**Malignant η = 77**	***P***
Palpable			**< 0,0001**
Palpable	79 (26,51 %)	58 (75 %)	
Not palpable	219(73,49%)	19 (25 %)	

2.2.2.1.1. Number

The total number of palpable masses was 137. The distribution of the number of masses (benign, malignant) per patient is shown in Table 18.

The vast majority of patients in our series had a palpable mass (93%).

Patients with benign masses were more likely to have multiple palpable masses than patients with malignant masses, with no significant difference (9.7% in the benign group vs. 3.6% in the malignant group;/; *= 0.18).*

Table 18. Distribution of the number of palpable masses per patient.			
Patient	**Benin n = 72**	**Malignant n = 56**	***P***
Number of masses per patient			0,15
1	65 (90,28 %)	54 (96,43 %)	
2	4 (5,56 %)	2 (3,57 %)	
3	3(4,17%)	0	

2.2.2.1.2. On the side

Of the 137 palpable masses, 69 were located in the right breast and 68 in the left. Malignant masses were more often located in the left breast compared with benign masses, but there was no significant difference (56.90% malignant masses vs 44.30% benign masses,^ = *0.14*) (table 19).

Table 19. Distribution of benign and malignant masses according side.			
Mass	**Benign η = 79**	**Malignant η = 58**	***P***
Visit			0,17
Right breast	44 (55,70 %)	25 (43,10 %)	
Left breast	35 (44,30 %)	33 (56,90 %)	

2.2.2.1.3. Seating by quadrant

One third of palpable masses (34.3%) were located in the upper exteme quadrant (37.97% of benign masses vs 29.31% of malignant masses,^= *0.29).* In addition, there were no masses located centrally, in the axillary extension or in the submammary sillum.

The quadrant distribution of benign and malignant masses is shown in Figure 19.

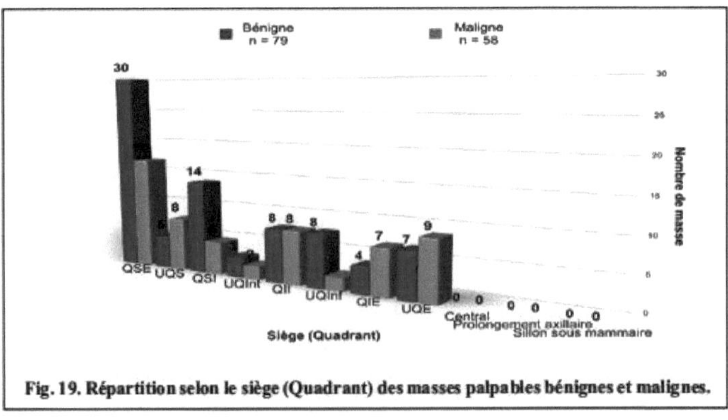

Fig. 19. Répartition selon le siège (Quadrant) des masses palpables bénignes et malignes.

Fig. 19. Quadrant distribution of palpable benign and malignant masses.

2.2.2.1.4. Size

The size of the palpable masses ranged from 10 to 120 mm, with an average of 28.59 + 14.17 mm.

The mean size of palpable benign and malignant masses was 27.63 + 15.35 mm (10-120 mm) and 29.91 + 12.41 mm (10-70 mm) respectively *(p = 0.33).*

The distribution of palpable masses by size, in 10 mm increments, shows a peak in the 20-30 mm range in both the benign and malignant groups combined (fig. 20).

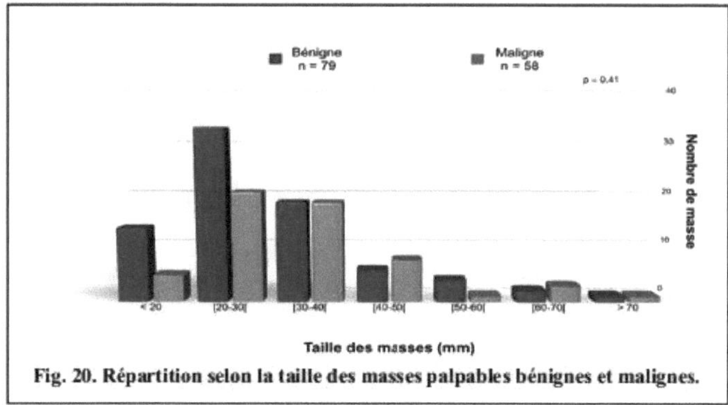

Fig. 20. Répartition selon la taille des masses palpables bénignes et malignes.

Fig. 20: Size distribution of palpable benign and malignant masses.

2.2.2.1.5. Mobility in relation to the superficial pian

115 palpable masses were mobile in relation to the superficial pian, of which 77 out of 79 were benign masses and 36 out of 58 malignant *masses (p<0, 0001).*

38% of malignant masses adhered to the superficial plane compared with 2.53% of benign masses *(p < 0.0001)* (table 20).

Table 20. Distribution of benign and malignant masses according to mobility in relation to the superficial plane.

Mass	Benign n = 79	Malignant n = 58	*P*
Mobility / surface plane			**< 0,0001**
Yes	77 (97,47 %)	36 (62 %)	
No	2 (2,53 %)	22 (38 %)	

2.2.2.1.6. Mobility in relation to the deep plane

116 palpable masses were mobile in relation to the deep plane, all benign masses and 37 out of 58 malignant masses 64% *(p < 0.0001)*

36% of malignant masses were deep-seated (table 21).

Table 21. Distribution of benign and malignant masses according to mobility in relation to the deep plane.

Mass	Benign n = 79	Malignant n = 58	*P*

Mobility/deep plane			**< 0,0001**
Yes	79 (100,00 %)	37 (64 %)	
No	0	21 (36%)	

2.2.2.1.7. Ganglion

None of the patients with benign masses axillary adenopathy on palpation, whereas 69% of patients with malignant masses had homolateral axillary adenopathy *($p < 0.0001$)*. There were no palpable contralateral axillary or supraclavicular adenopathies.

3. Imaging features

3.2. Mammography

Mammography was performed in 256 patients, in all patients a malignant lesion (72 patients) and in 184 of the 258 patients with a benign lesion, most often as part of screening. In the case of the 74 patients with benign lesions who had not undergone mammography, their young age did not allow them to undergo this examination.

3.2.2. Breast density

The distribution according to breast density of patients in the benign and malignant groups is shown in Table 22 and Figure 21.

Table 22. Distribution according to breast density of patients in the benign and malignant groups.

Patient	Benin n=184	Malignant n=72	*P*
Breast density			0,002
a	24 (13,04 %)	24 (33,33 %)	
b	90 (48,91 %)	29 (40,28 %)	
c	61 (33,15 %)	15 (20,83 %)	
d	9 (4,89 %)	4 (5,56 %)	

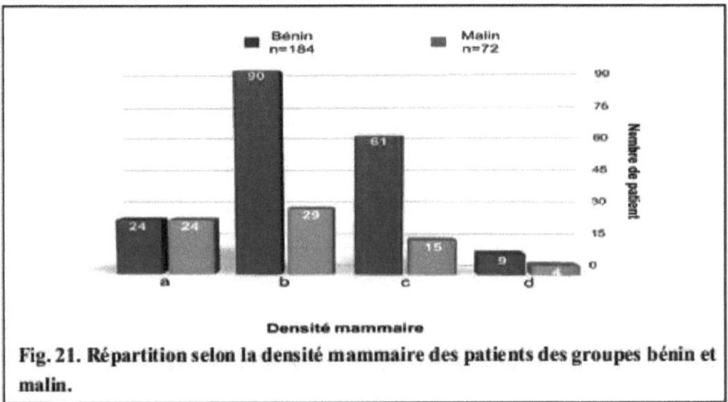

Fig. 21. Répartition selon la densité mammaire des patients des groupes bénin et malin.

Fig. 21: Distribution of patients in the benign and malignant groups according to breast density.

Patients with benign masses had denser breasts, often of types b and c (82.1%) than patients with malignant lesions, often of types a and b (73.6%) *(p = 0.002).*

3.2.3. Mass

3.2.3.1. Visibility

On mammography, 164 masses out of 281 were visible (58.36%). Some patients had more than one mass.

Malignant masses were more often visible on mammography than benign masses, respectively 90% vs 46.57%,j9 < *0.0001* (table 23).

Table 23. Distribution according to the visibility of the mass on mammography.

Mass	**Benign n = 204**	**Malignant n = 77**	***P***
Mass visibility			**< 0,0001**
Yes	95 (46,57 %)	**69 (90 %)**	
No	109 (53,43 %)	**8 (10%)**	

3.2.3.2. Visit

Of the 164 masses visible on mammography, 85 masses (51.89%) were located in the right breast and 79 masses (48.17%) in the left breast. Malignant masses were more often visible in the left breast than benign masses (59.42% malignant masses vs 40% benign masses, *p = 0.014*) (table 24).

Table 24. Distribution according to site of benign and malignant masses visible on mammography.

Patient	**Benign η = 95**	**Malignant η = 69**	***P***
Visit			**0,014**
Right breast	57 (60%)	28 (40,58 %)	
Left breast	38 (40 %)	41 (59,42 %)	

3.2.3.3. Seating by quadrant

39.02% of the masses visible on mammography were located in the upper extremity quadrant (43.16% of benign masses vs 33.33% of malignant masses,^ = *0.08).*

The distribution of benign and malignant masses visible on mammography by site (quadrant) is shown in Figure 22.

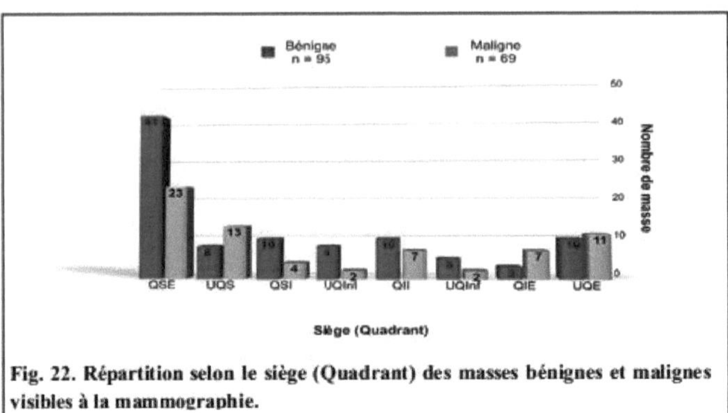

Fig. 22. Répartition selon le siège (Quadrant) des masses bénignes et malignes visibles à la mammographie.

Fig. 22. Quadrant distribution of benign and malignant masses visible on mammosranchia.

3.2.3.4. Breast area

Malignant masses were often found in the posterior third of the gland (52.17%) and exceptionally in the anterior third (13.04%) *($p < 0.000001$)*. Benign masses were often found in the middle mammary region (44.21%) (table 25).

Table 25. Distribution of masses visible on mammography according to breast area.

Mass	**Benign n = 95**	**Malignant n = 69**	***P***
Breast area			**0,008**
Front	25 (26,32 %)	9(13,04%)	
Average	42 (44,21 %)	24 (34,78 %)	
Posterior	28 (29,47 %)	36 (52,17%)	

3.2.3.5. Size

The average size of the masses visible on mammography was 25.91 + 15.11 mm, with extremes ranging from 5 mm to 88 mm.

The mean size of malignant masses visible on mammography was greater than that of benign masses, respectively 31.7 + 17.05 mm (5-88 mm) and 21.72 ± 11.96 mm (7-67 mm) *($p < 0.0001$)*.

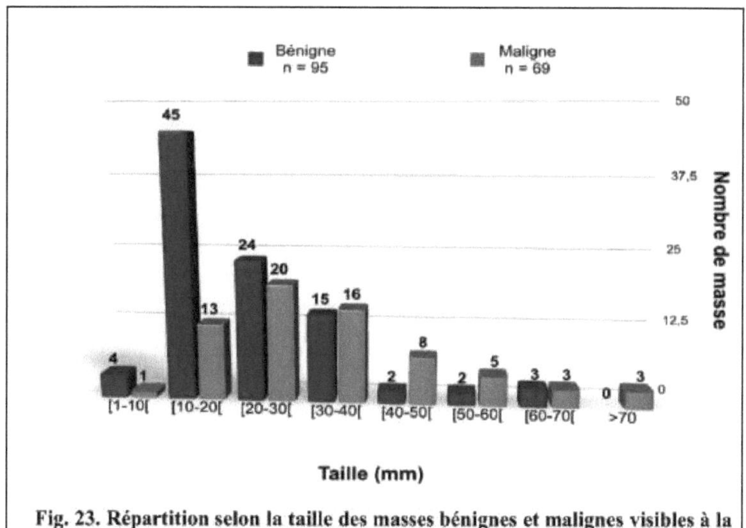

Fig. 23. Répartition selon la taille des masses bénignes et malignes visibles à la mammographie.

The distribution of masses visible on mammography according to size, by 10 mm bands, shows a peak in the 20-30 mm band in the group of malignant masses and in the 10-20 mm band in the group of benign masses (fig. 23).

3.2.3.6. Distance from nipple

The mean distance of the benign and malignant masses visible on mammography from the nipple was 56.28 + 33.64 mm (0-196 mm) and 57.88 + 34.llmm (0-139 mm) respectively *(p = 0.53)*.

3.2.3.7. Mass characteristics

3.1.2.7.1. Shape

As shown in Table 26, benign masses were in the vast majority of cases oval in shape (81.05%) and rarely irregular (8.42%*) (p < 0.0001)*, unlike malignant masses which were often irregular (86.96%) and exceptionally oval (4.35%) *(p < 0.0001)*.

Table 26. Distribution according to shape of masses visible on mammography.

Mass	**Benign n = 95**	**Malignant n = 69**	***P***
Shape of the mass			**< 0,0001**
Oval	77 (81,05 %)	3 (4,35 %)	
Round	10 (10,53 %)	6 (8,70 %)	
Irregular	8 (8,42 %)	60 (86,96 %)	

3.1.2.7.2. Contours

On mammography, benign masses were most often circumscribed or masked in outline (76.84%,j9 < *0.0001*). Malignant masses, on the other hand, were often indistinct and spiculated in outline (82.61%,p< *0.0001).*

The distribution of benign and malignant masses visible on mammography is shown in table 27.

Table 27. Distribution according to contour of masses visible on mammography.			
Mass	**Benign n = 95**	**Malignant n = 69**	*P*
Contours of the mass			**< 0,0001**
Circumscribed	32 (33,68 %)	0	
Masked	41 (43,16%)	8(11,59%)	
Microlobulations	18(18,95%)	4 (5,80 %)	
Indistinct	4 (4,21 %)	20 (28,99 %)	
Spiculated	0	37 (53,62 %)	

3.1.2.7.3. Density

Table 28 summarises the density of benign and malignant masses on mammography, and shows that the vast majority of benign masses were isodense in relation to the gland (84.42%, $p < 0.0001$). Malignant masses were more often hyperdense in relation to the gland (94.20%,j9 < *0.0001).*

Furthermore, we did not note any calcium mass in our series.

Table 28. Distribution according to density of benign and malignant masses visible on mammography.			
Mass	**Benign n = 95**	**Malignant n = 69**	***P***
Mass			**< 0,0001**
Hypodense	1 (1,05 %)	0	
fsodense	84 (88,42 %)	4 (5,80 %)	
Hyperdense	9 (9,47 %)	65 (94,20 %)	
Calcium	0	0	
Grease gun	1 (1,05 %)	0	

3.1.2.7.4. Associated signs

The results of the analysis of signs associated with benign and malignant masses on mammography are shown in tables 29 and 30. Associated signs were noted in 37 out of 281 mammograms performed, i.e. 13.17%. In most cases (33/281), they were associated with malignant masses and only 4 cases were associated with benign masses. These associated signs included microcalcifications, skin thickening, skin and nipple retractions and axillary adenopathies.

Microcalcifications were visible only in cases of malignant masses (13/33 of cases, 39.39%). These microcalcifications were more often fine and pleomorphic (7 cases), coarse or heterogenous in 3 cases, two cases of amorphous calcifications and in one case they were fine and linear, or even branched. The distribution of microcalcifications on mammography was often grouped in clusters (8 cases) or segmental (5 cases).

Skin thickening was observed in 3 cases of benign lesions and 3 cases of malignant lesions *(p<0, 0001).*

Skin retraction was found in 8 cases of malignant lesions and one case of benign lesions (p < 0.001).

Nipple retraction and axillary adenopathy on mammography were only associated with malignant masses in 9 and 13 cases respectively.

Furthermore, we did not note architectural distortion or asymmetry of density in our series.

Table 29. Distribution according to signs associated with masses visible on mammography.

Mass	**Benign n = 204**	**Malignant n = 77**	***P***
Associated signs			**< 0,0001**
Yes	4(1,96%)	33 (43 %)	
No	200 (98,04 %)	44 (57 %)	

Table 30. Distribution according to the type of signs associated with masses visible on mammography.

Patient	**Benin n = 4**	**Malin n = 33**	***P***
Types of associated signs			
Microcalcifications	0	13 (23,21 %)	**< 0,0001**
Architectural distortion	0	0	1
Density asymmetry	0	0	1
Skin thickening	3 (75 %)	13 (23,21 %)	**0,000016**
Skin retraction	1 (15 %)	8(14,29%)	**0,000003**
Nipple retraction	0	9 (16,07 %)	**0,00005**
Axillary nodes	0	13 (23,21 %)	**< 0,0001**

3.1.3. ACR BI-RADS category

More than half of the mammograms performed were classified BI-RADS 0 (59.1%), 75% of the masses were benign and only 16.88% were malignant,^ < *0.0001.*

The distribution of benign and malignant masses according to mammographic BI-RADS is summarised in table 31.

Table 31. Distribution of benign and malignant masses according to mammographic BI-RADS.

Mass	**Benign n = 204**	**Malignant n = 77**	***P***
BI-RADS category for mammography			**< 0,0001**
0	153 (75,00 %)	13 (16,88 %)	
3	26 (12,75 %)	0	
4a	18(8,82%)	3 (3,90 %)	

4b	1 (0,49 %)	2 (2,60 %)	
4c	6 (2,94 %)	16 (20,78 %)	
5	0	43 (55,84 %)	

3.2. Ultrasound

The total number of masses found on ultrasound was 375, including 298 benign masses (79.46%) and 77 malignant masses (20.53%).

Four patients had two or more multicentric malignant masses.

3.2.2. Breast ultrasound

In our series, 60.30% of patients had a heterogeneous breast echotexture (fatty and glandular), 64.34% of patients in the benign group and 45.83% of patients in the malignant group *(p = 0.005).*

The distribution of patients according to breast echostructure is shown in Table 32.

Table 32. Distribution according breast echotexture of benign and malignant patients.

Patient	**Benin n=258**	**Malignant n=72**	***P***
Breast ultrasound			**< 0,0001**
a	42 (16,28 %)	31 (43,06 %)	
b	50 (19,38 %)	8(11,11 %)	
c	166 (64,34 %)	33 (45,83 %)	

3.2.3. Mass

3.2.3.7. Visit

On ultrasound, of the 375 masses, 189 (50.4%) were located in left breast and 186 (49.6%) in the right breast (p = 0.83).

Malignant masses were often located in the left breast (57.14% malignant masses vs 48.66% benign masses, but with no significant difference, *p = 0.18*) (table 33).

Table 33. Distribution of benign and malignant masses according to site.

Mass	**Benign n = 298**	**Malignant n = 77**	***P***
Visit			**0,20**
Right breast	153 (51,34 %)	33 (42,86 %)	
Left breast	145 (48,66 %)	44 (57,14 %)	

3.2.3.8. Seating by quadrant

Half of the masses in our series (50.13%) were located in the upper quadrant and at the union of the outer quadrants (50.7% of benign masses vs 48.05% of malignant masses,^ = *0.68).*

The quadrant distribution of benign and malignant masses is shown in Figure 24.

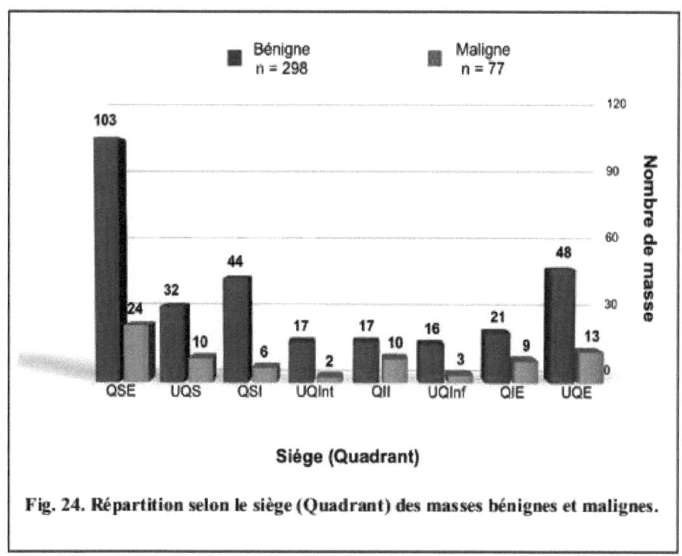

Fig. 24. Répartition selon le siège (Quadrant) des masses bénignes et malignes.

Fig. 24. Quadrant distribution benign and malignant masses.

3.2.3.9. Size

The mean ultrasound mass size was 19.12 + 11.15 mm, with extremes ranging from 4.8 mm to 12 mm.

The mean size of malignant masses on ultrasound was greater than that of benign masses, respectively 24.46 + 11.53 mm (6-59 mm) and 17.74 + 10.64 mm (4.8-112 mm) *($p < 0.0001$).*

The distribution of masses on ultrasound according to size, by 10 mm bands, shows a peak in the 10-20 mm band in the benign and malignant groups (fig. 25).

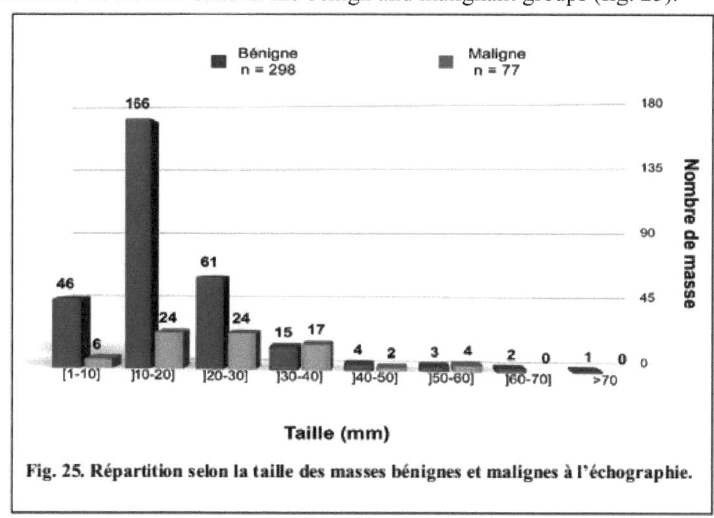

Fig. 25. Répartition selon la taille des masses bénignes et malignes à l'échographie.

Fig. 25. Size distribution of benign and malignant masses on ultrasound.

3.2.3.10. Distance from nipple

The mean distance of the masses from the nipple on ultrasound was 42.26 + 23.16 mm, with extremes ranging from 0 mm to 27 mm.

The mean distance of the benign and malignant masses from the nipple on ultrasound was 41.50 + 21.88 mm (1.8-108 mm) and 45.20 + 27.52 mm (0-127 mm) respectively *(p = 0.2 7).*

3.2.3.11. Distance from skin

The mean distance of the masses from the skin on ultrasound was 8.11+5.29 mm, with extremes ranging from 0 mm to 31.7 mm.

The mean distance of the benign and malignant masses from the skin on ultrasound was 8.33 + 5.43 mm (0-31.7 mm) and 7.27 + 4.63 mm (0-21.2 mm) respectively (p = 0.08).

3.2.3.12. Breast thickness

In our series, the mean breast thickness on ultrasound was 36.07 + 15.20 mm, with extremes ranging from 9 mm to 117 mm.

The mean thickness of the breast on ultrasound in the malignant group was greater, 38.02 + 13.26 mm, than in the benign group, 35.57 + 15.64 mm, but with no significant difference (p = 0.16).

3.2.3.13. Mass characteristics

3.2.3.13.1. Shape

On ultrasound, the vast majority of benign masses were oval in shape (86.24%) and rarely irregular (8.05%) *(p < 0.0001).* In contrast, malignant masses were often irregular (88.31%) and rarely oval (6.49%) *(p<0.0001)* at .

The distribution of benign and malignant masses on ultrasound is shown in table 34.

Table 34. Distribution of benign and malignant masses on ultrasound according to shape

Mass	**Benign n = 298**	**Malignant n = 77**	***P***
Shape			**< 0,0001**
Oval	**257 (86,24 %)**	**5 (6,49 %)**	
Round	**17(5,70%)**	**4(5,19%)**	
Irregular	**24 (8,05 %)**	**68 (88,31 %)**	

1.1.1.1.1. Orientation

As shown in Table 35, benign masses were more often parallel to the skin (97.65%*) (p < 0.0001).* Unlike malignant masses, which were often not parallel to the skin (79.22%) *(p < 0.0001).*

Table 35. Distribution according to orientation of benign and malignant

masses on ultrasound.			
Mass	**Benign n = 298**	**Malignant n = 77**	***P***
Orientation			**< 0,0001**
Parallel to the skin	291 (97,65 %)	16 (20,78 %)	
Not parallel to the skin	7 (2,35 %)	61 (79,22 %)	

3.2.2.7.3. Contours

On ultrasound, benign masses were most often circumscribed or microlobulated (96.3%, *p < 0.0001*). Conversely, malignant masses were often angular and spiculated (81.8%,^ *< 0.0001).*

The distribution of benign and malignant masses on ultrasound is shown in table 36.

Table 36. Contour distribution of benign and malignant masses on ultrasound.			
Mass	**Benign n = 298**	**Malignant n = 77**	***P***
Contours			**< 0,0001**
Circumscribed	88 (29,53 %)	0	
Microlobulated	199 (66,78 %)	8(10,39%)	
Indistinct	9 (3,02 %)	6 (7,79 %)	
Angular	2 (0,67 %)	19 (24,68 %)	
Spiculated	0	44 (57,14 %)	

3.2.2.7.4. Border

As shown in Table 37, benign masses were more often thin-edged (96.64%*) (p < 0.0001).* In contrast, malignant masses often had a peripheral echogenic halo (67.53%*) (p < 0.0001).*

Table 37. Distribution according to border of benign and malignant masses on ultrasound.			
Mass	**Benign n = 298**	**Malignant n = 77**	***P***
Border			**< 0,0001**
Fine	288 (96,64 %)	25 (32,47 %)	
Echogenic halo	10 (3,36 %)	52 (67,53 %)	

3.2.2.7.5. Echostructure

Table 38 summarises the echostructure of benign and malignant masses on ultrasound, showing that the vast majority of benign masses were isoechoic or hypoechoic to fat (95%. y< *0.0001*). On the other hand, malignant masses were more often hypoechoic to fat (92.21%,y< *0.0001).*

No anechogenic masses were found in our series.

Table 38. Distribution according to echostructure of benign and malignant masses on ultrasound.

Mass	Benign n = 298	Malignant n = 77	*P*
Echostructure			**< 0,0001**
Anechogenic	**0**	**0**	
Isoechogenic	130 (43,62 %)	**0**	
Hypoechoic	153 (51,34 %)	71 (92,21 %)	
Hyperechoic	2 (0,67 %)	**0**	
Complex	12 (4,03 %)	**3 (3,90 %)**	
Heterogeneous	1 (0,34 %)	**3 (3,90 %)**	

1.1.1.1.1. Posterior acoustic signs

On ultrasound, the vast majority of benign masses showed no posterior acoustic signs (90.9%, *p < 0.0001*). Conversely, malignant masses were often attenuating (57.14%, p < *0.0001).*

The distribution according to posterior acoustic signs of benign and malignant masses on ultrasound is shown in table 39.

Table 39. Distribution according to posterior acoustic signs of benign and malignant masses on ultrasound.

Mass	Benign n = 298	Malignant n = 77	*P*
Posterior acoustic signs			
No effect	**271 (90,94 %)**	**28 (36,36 %)**	**< 0,0001**
Reinforcement	**13 (4,36%)**	**3 (3,90 %)**	**0,89**
Attenuation	**8 (2,68 %)**	**44 (57,14 %)**	**< 0,0001**
Combined	**6 (2,01 %)**	**2 (2,60 %)**	**0,90**

3.2.2.7.7. Calcifications

Of the 375 masses studied 81 or 21.6% had calcifications visible on ultrasound (40 out of 77 [51.95%] malignant masses and 41 out of 298 [13.76%] benign masses,^ < *0.0001*) (table 40).

We note that the calcifications are all located in the masses on ultrasound.

Table 40. Distribution according to the presence of calcifications in benign and malignant masses on ultrasound.

Mass	Benign η = 298	Malignant η = 77	*P*
Calcifications			**0,0001**
Absent	257 (86,24 %)	37 (48,05 %)	
Present	41 (13,76%)	40 (51,95 %)	

3.2.2.7.8. Colour Doppler vascularisation

Of the 375 masses in our series, 309 (82.4%) were vascularised on colour Doppler, 235 (78.86%) benign masses versus 74 (96.1%) malignant masses *(p = 0.0004).*

There was an absence of vascularisation of malignant masses in three cases (3.9%) compared with 63 (21.14%) benign masses *(p = 0.0004).*

Table 41 shows that strong vascularisation (central and peripheral) was more frequently observed in malignant masses than in benign masses (66.23% vs 32.21%,^ < 0.0001).

Table 41. Distribution according to vascularisation of benign and malignant masses on colour Doppler.			
Mass	**Benign n = 298**	**Malignant n = 77**	***P***
Vascularisation			**< 0,0001**
Absent	63 (21,14%)	3 (3,90%)	
Peripheral	135 (45,30 %)	16 (20,78 %)	
Central	4(1,34%)	7 (9,09 %)	
Central and peripheral	96 (32,21 %)	51 (66,23 %)	

3.2.2.7.9. Associated signs

The results of the analysis of signs associated with benign and malignant masses on ultrasound are shown in tables 42 and 43.

Associated signs were often found in malignant cases (29.87%) and rarely in benign cases (1.34%*) (p < 0.0001).*

These associated signs corresponded to echogenic galactophoric ectasia, skin thickening, skin and nipple retraction as well as rndema and hypervascularisation of the surrounding tissue.

Skin thickening was associated with benign lesions in 2 cases and malignant lesions in 8 cases *(p < 0.0001).*

Skin retraction was found in 10 cases of malignant lesions and one case of benign lesion *(p < 0.0001).*

Rndema of the surrounding tissue was found in 12 cases of malignant lesions and one case of benign lesion *(p < 0.0001).*

Echogenic galatophoric ectasia, nipple retraction and hypervascularisation of the surrounding tissue on colour Doppler were associated only with malignant masses, in 2, 7 and 11 cases respectively.

In our series, there was no architectural distortion or invasion of the pectoralis muscle.

Table 42. Distribution according associated signs of benign and malignant masses on ultrasound.			
Mass	**Benign n = 298**	**Malignant n = 77**	***P***
Associated signs			**< 0,0001**
Absence	294 (98,87 %)	54 (70,13 %)	
Presence	4(1,34%)	23 (29,87 %)	

Table 43. Distribution according to the type of associated signs of benign and malignant masses on ultrasound.			
Mass	**Benign η = 4**	**Malignant η = 23**	***P***

Types of associated signs			
Architectural distortion	0	0	1
Echogenic galactophoric ectasia	0	2	0,06
Skin thickening	2	8	**< 0,0001**
Skin retraction	1	10	**< 0,0001**
Nipple retraction	0	**7**	**< 0,0001**
ffidema	1	12	**< 0,0001**
Hypervascularisation	0	11	**< 0,0001**
Invasion of the pectoral muscle	0	0	1

3.2.2.7.10. Ganglion

On ultrasound, 61 patients had adenopathies, 59 out of 72 (81.94%) in the malignant group and 2 out of 258 (0.008%) in the benign group *(p<0.0001).*

The distribution of benign and malignant masses on ultrasound according to lymph node involvement is shown in table 44.

Table 44. Distribution according to lymph node involvement of patients in the benign and malignant groups on ultrasound.

Patient	**Benin n = 258**	**Malignant n = 72**	***P***
Nodes			
Homolateral	2	55	**< 0,0001**
Peripheral axillae	2	58	**< 0,0001**
Central axillae	0	12	**< 0,0001**
Subclavicular	0	4	**< 0,0001**
Internal mammary	0	0	1
Sus clavicularis	0	0	1
Controlateral	0	1	0,06

3.2.2.7.11. ACR BI-RADS category

The results of the ultrasound BI-RADS classification in our series were 76 masses (20.27%) classified as BI-RADS 3, 192 masses (51.2%) classified as BIRADS 4a, 11 masses (2.93%) classified as BI-RADS 4b, 41 masses classified as BIRADS 4c and 55 masses (14.67%) classified as BI-RADS 5.

The distribution of benign and malignant masses according to the BI-RADS classification is shown in table 45.

Table 45. Distribution according to BI-RADS classification of benign and malignant masses on ultrasound.

Mass	**Benign n = 298**	Malignant n = 77	**Percentage of malignancy**	***P***
BI-RADS category				**< 0,0001**
3	76 (25,50%)	0	0	

4a	190 (63,76%)	2 (2,60%)	1,04%	
4b	7 (2,35%)	4(5,19%)	36,36%	
4c	23 (7,72%)	18 (23,38%)	43,90%	
5	2 (0,67%)	53 (68,83 %)	96%	

Among the benign lesions, 76 masses (25.50%) were classified BI-RADS 3 and 222 masses (74.50%) were classified BI-RADS 4a, 4b, 4and 5.
All malignant masses were classified as BI-RADS 4a, 4b, 4c and 5; no mass was classified as BIRADS 3.
We have noted that the proportion of malignant lesions increases with the BI-RADS 4 sub-categories a, b, c.

3.3. Elastography

3.3.1. Quality parameters

3.3.1.1. Consistent colour cartography

Most of the masses were not very homogeneous (71.47%) (Fig. 26). In fact, the colour mapping was not very homogeneous in two thirds of the benign masses and in half of the malignant masses (Table 46).

able 46. Distribution according homogeneity of colour mapping of benign and malignant masses on elastography.

Mass	**Benign n = 298**	**Malignant n = 77**	***P***
Consistent mapping			**< 0,0001**
Homogenous	17(5,70%)	18 (23,38 %)	
Not very homogeneous	228 (76,51 %)	40 (51,95 %)	
Heterogeneous	53 (17,79 %)	19 (24,68 %)	

Fig. 26: Inconsistent flow maps (a) Fibroadenoma (b) NST infiltrating ductal carcinoma.

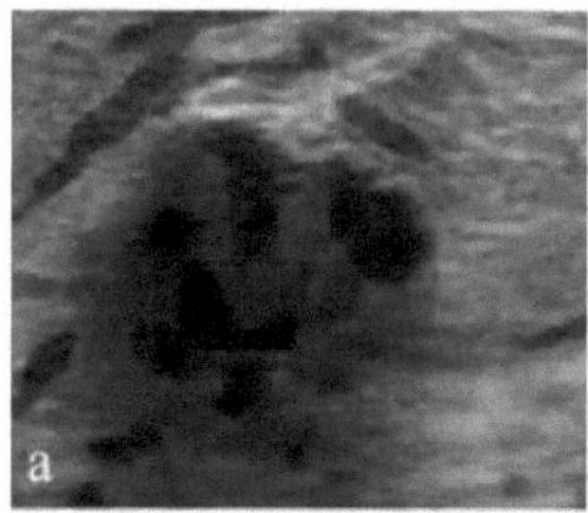

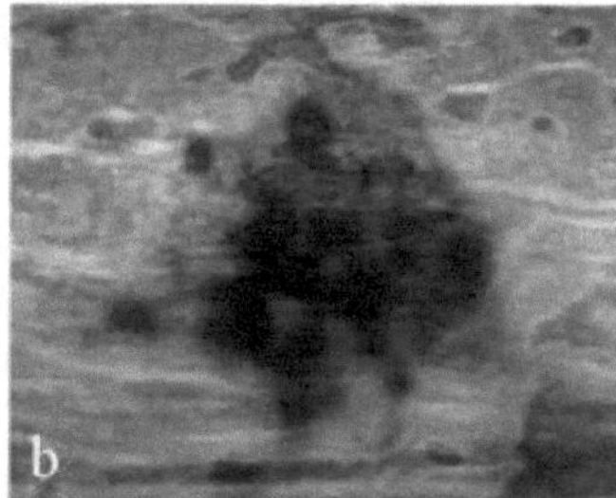

3.3.1.2. Maximum cartographic colour

On elastography, the maximum colour of benign masses was green (intermediate component) in the vast majority of cases (74.16%,ρ< *0.0001)* and blue (hard component) in malignant masses (96.10%,^ < *0.0001*) (fig. 27).
The distribution according to maximum colour of the mapping of benign and

malignant masses on elastography is shown in Table 47.

Table 47. Distribution according to maximum colour of the mapping of benign and malignant masses on elastography.

Mass	Benign n = 298	Malignant n = 77	*P*
Maximum mapping colour			< 0,0001
Red (flexible component)	2 (0,67 %)	**0**	
Green (intermediate component)	221 (74,16%)	**3 (3,90 %)**	
Blue (hard component)	75 (25,17 %)	74 **(96,10 %)**	

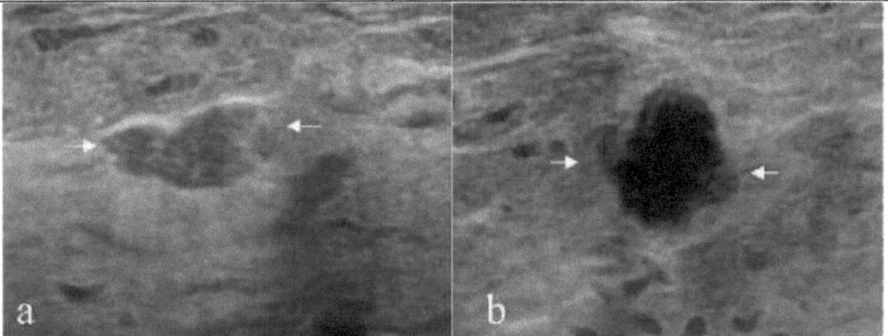

Fig. 27: Maximum colour on mapping: (a) Mass whose maximum colour was green (arrows). Fibroadenoma. (b) Mass whose maximum colour was blue (arrows). Papillary carcinoma.

3.3.1.3. Location the hardest area

The hardest area on elastography for benign masses was most often peri-lesional (76.83%,j9 < *0.0001*). For malignant lesions, the hardest area on mapping was intra- and peri-lesional (81.82%, p < *0.0001*) (table 48) (fig. 28).

Table 48. Distribution according to the location the hardest zone of benign and malignant masses on elastography.

Mass	Benign n = 298	Malignant n = 77	*P*
Location the hardest area			
Intra-lesional	74 (24,83 %)	13 (16,88 %)	0,14
Lesion perimeter	220 (73,83 %)	1 (1,30%)	**< 0,0001**
Intra- and peri-injury	4(1,34%)	63 (81,82 %)	**< 0,0001**

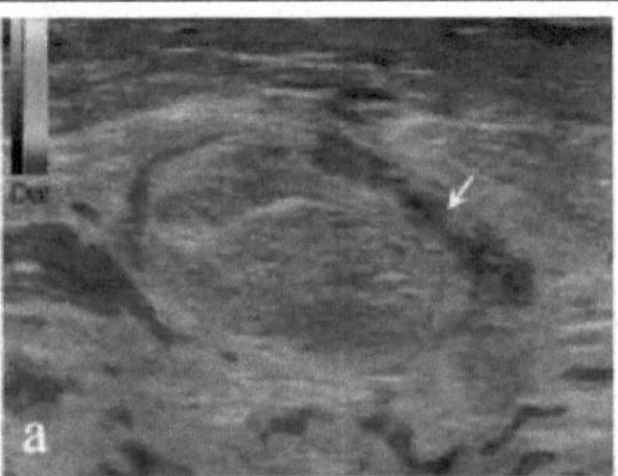

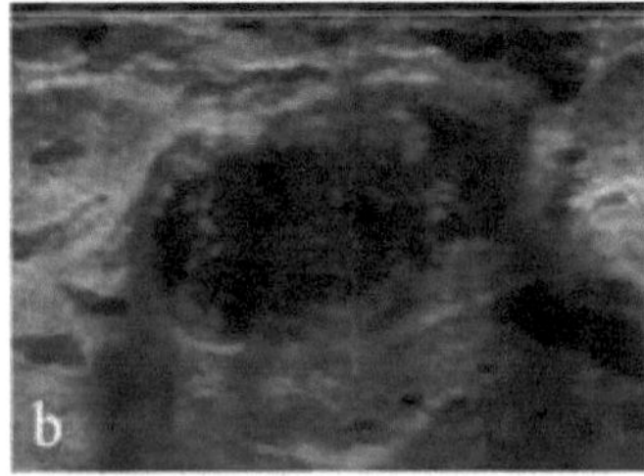

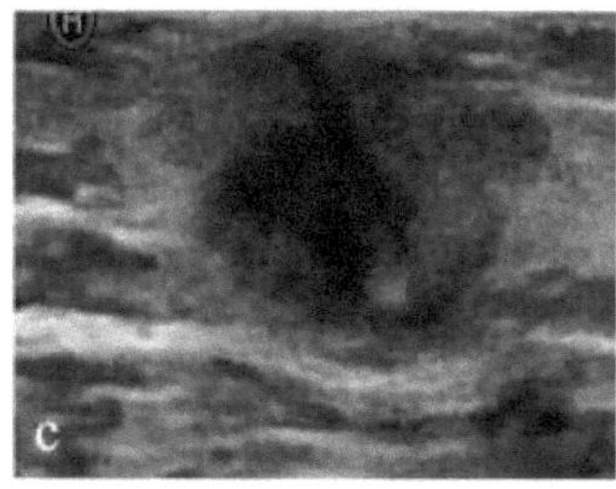

Fig. 28: Location the hardest zone on elastography.
(a) Peri lesion (arrow). Fibroadenoma. (b) Intra-lesional. Phyllodes tumour, (c) Peri- and intra-lesional. NST infiltrating carcinoma.

3.3.1.4. Toxic lesion

98.4% of masses showed intra-lesional echoes (99.66% benign lesions vs 93.51% malignant lesions).
Lesions with an echo void on colour mapping are often malignant *($p < 0.0001$)* (table 49) (fig. 29).

Table 49. Distribution according to the presence of intra-lesional echo of benign and malignant masses on elastography.

Mass	Benign n = 298	Malignant n = 77	*P*
Intra-lesional ultrasound			**0,0009**
Presence	297 (99,66%)	72 (93,51%)	
Empty echo	1 (0,34%)	**5 (6,49%)**	

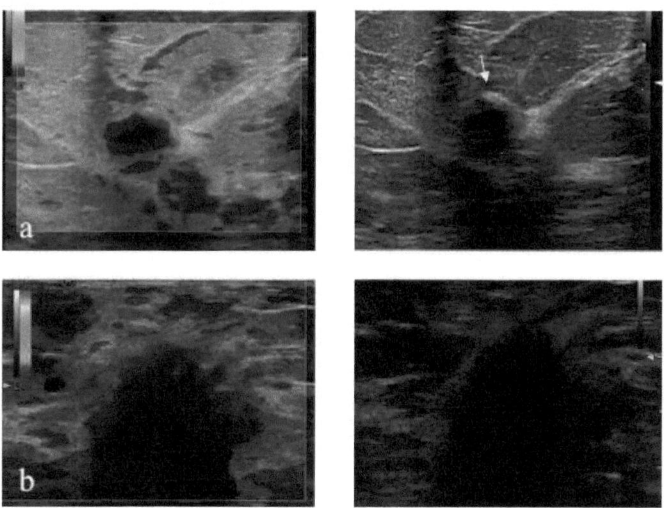

Fig. 29: Intra-lesion echo void on colour mapping. Elastographic images and corresponding ultrasound images. (a) Remodeled cyst, parietal calcification (arrow). (b) NST infiltrating carcinoma.

3.3.1.5. Colorimetric score

Among the 375 masses classified by colorimetric score, score 1 in 10 cases (2.67%), score 2 in 213 cases (56.8%), score 3 in 76 cases (20.27%), score 4 in 9 cases (2.4%) and score 5 in 67 cases (17.87%). In total, scores 1, 2 and 3, considered benign, represented 299 cases, or 79.73% of the total, and scores 4 and 5, considered malignant, represented 76 cases, or 20.26% of the total (fig. 30).

The distribution according to the colorimetric score of benign and malignant masses on elastography is shown in table 50.

Table 50. Distribution according to colorimetric score of benign and malignant masses on elastography.

Mass	**Benign n = 298**	**Malignant n = 77**	*P*
Colorimetric score			**< 0,0001**
1	10 (3,36 %)	**0**	
2	212(71,14 %)	1 (1,30%)	
3	69 (23,15 %)	7 (9,09 %)	
4	3 (1,01 %)	6 (7,79 %)	
5	4(1,34 %)	63 (81,82 %)	

Seven masses (2.35%) with a score considered malignant (score 4 and 5) were histologically benign.

Eight masses (10.39%) with a score considered benign (score 1, 2 and 3) turned out to be malignant.

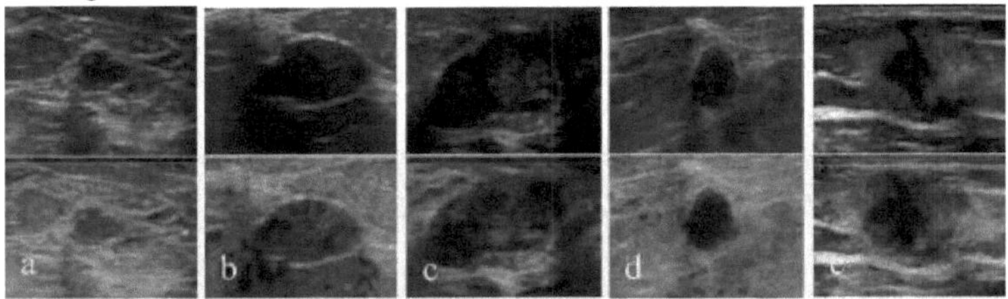

Fig. 30: Elasticity score. Elastographic images and corresponding ultrasound images. (a) Score 1: Fibroadenoma, (b) Score 2: Fibroadenoma, (c) Score 3: Phyllodes tumour, (d) Score 4: Papillary carcinoma. (e) Score 5: Invasive carcinomaNST.

3.3.2. Quantitative parameters

3.3.2.1. Elasticity ratio

3.3.2.1.1. Grease-to-injury ratio

In the 375 masses, the mean fat-to-lesion ratio on elastography was 8.36 + 21.86, with extremes ranging from 0.62 to 217.7.

The mean fat-to-lesion ratio in the group of malignant masses on elastography was 32.7 + 39.89 (2.66-217.7) higher than in the group of benign masses 2.1 + 1.18 (0.62-13), very significantly ($p < 0.0001$) (fig.31).

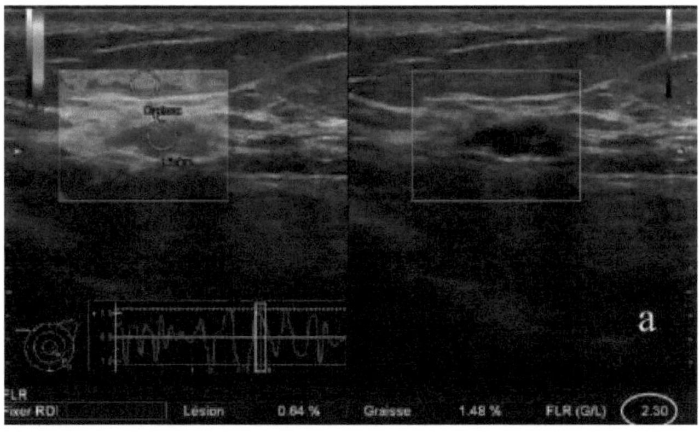

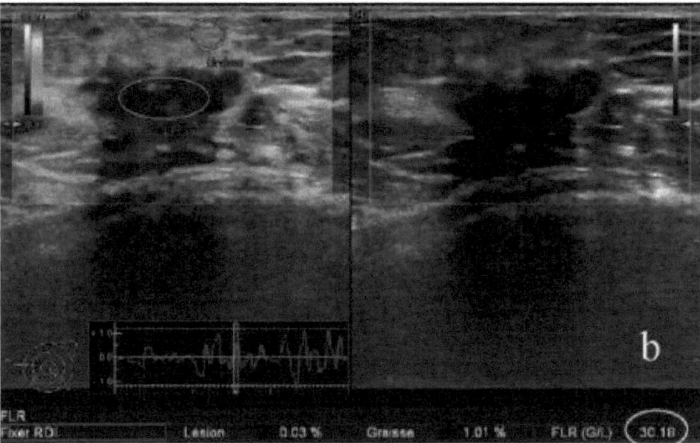

Fig. 31: Fat-to-injury ratio. (a) Elasticity ratio calculated at 2.3. Fibrocystic mastopathy (b) Elasticity ratio calculated at 30.18. Invasive carcinomaNST.

3.3.2.1.2. Gland-to-lesion ratio

Of the 375 masses, the gland-lesion ratio was only achieved for 315 masses, i.e. 84%, due to the absence of glandular tissue on the elastographic image.

The mean gland-to-lesion ratio on elastography was 6.13 + 2.68, with extremes ranging from 0.08 to 77.

The mean gland-to-lesion ratio in the group of elastographically malignant masses was 8.98 + 13.79 (0.68 - 77) higher than in the group of benign masses 1.5 + 0.67 (0.08 - 5.46), significantly so ($p < 0.0001$) (fig. 32).

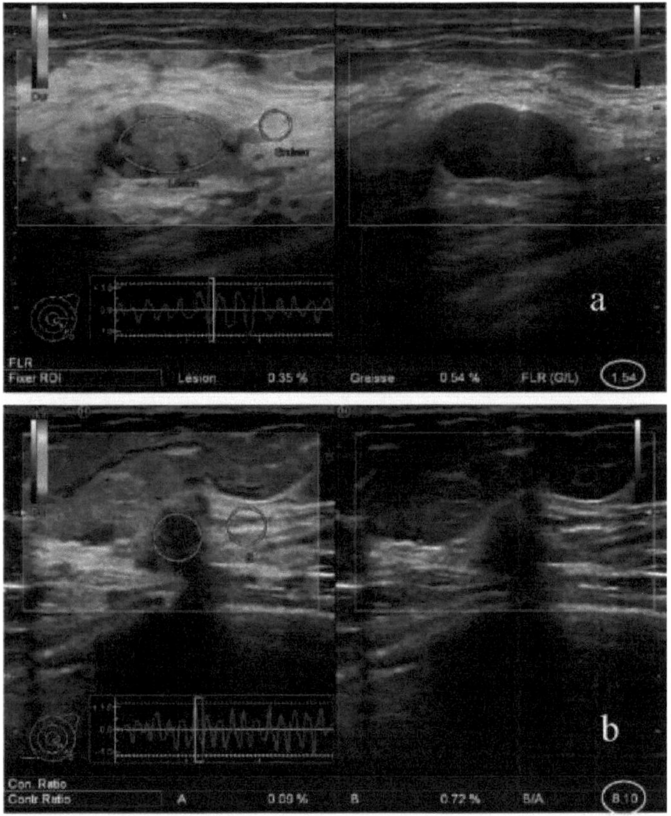

Fig. 32: Gland-to-lesion ratio. (a) Elasticity ratio calculated at 1.54. Fibroadenoma. Fibroadenoma (b) Elasticity ratio calculated at 8.10. NST infllrant carcinoma.

3.3.2.2. Size ratio

The mean elastographic size ratio of the 375 masses was 1.04 + 0.15, with extremes ranging from 0.76 to 2.27.

The mean size ratio of malignant masses on elastography was 1.23 + 0.22 (1-2.27) higher than that of benign masses 0.99 + 0.05 (0.76 - 1.45), significantly *so (p < 0.0001)* (fig.33).

In benign tumours, the size ratio was in the vast majority of cases less than or equal to 1 (96.98%,^ < *0.0001*). Conversely, for malignant tumours, the size ratio was often greater than 1 (89.61%,^ < *0.0001*) (table 51).

Table 51. Distribution according to size ratio of benign and malignant masses on elastography.

Mass	Benign n = 298	Malignant n = 77	*P*
Size ratio			**< 0,0001**
< 1	289 (96,98 %)	8(10,39%)	

> 1	9 (3,02%)	69 (89,61 %)	

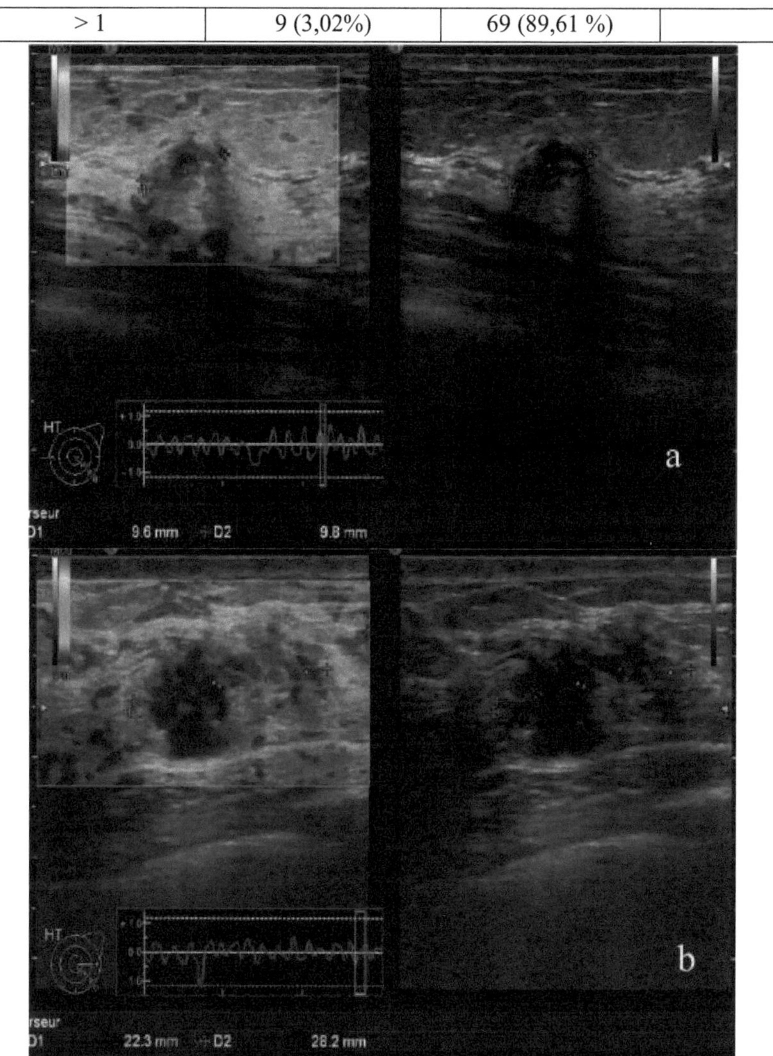

Fig. 33: Size ratio (a) Size ratio calculated at 0.98. Fibroadenoma. Fibroadenoma (b) Size ratio calculated at 1.26. NST infllrant carcinoma.

4. Histological characteristics

4.1. Results of ultrasound-guided biopsies

All the masses studied underwent percutaneous biopsy for histological correlation, 352 microbiopsies and 23 macrobiopsies under ultrasound.

The average number of samples was 5.93 + 1.85 cores per mass (2 toll cores).

Anatomopathological examination of the 375 masses revealed 298 (79.47%) benign masses and 77 (20.05%) malignant masses.

4.1.1. Benign lesions

Among the benign lesions, pathological analysis revealed 189 fibroadenomas (63.42%), 30 low-grade phyllodes tumours (10.07%), 55 fibrocystic mastopathies (18.46%), 4 adenomyepitheliomas (1.34%), 3 papillomas (1,01%), and 17 (5.7%) miscellaneous lesions (5 granulomatous mastitis, 3 cytosteatonecrosis, 2 reworked cysts, 2 galactophoritis, 2 pseudoangiomatous stremal hyperplasia, an epidermal cyst, an abscess and a lymph node) (table 52 and fig. 34).

Table 52. Distribution of benign lesions according to biopsy results.

Mass	**Benign η = 298**
Benign lesions	
Adenofibroma	189 (63,42 %)
Low-grade phyllodes tumour	30 (10,07 %)
Fibrocystic mastopathy	55 (18,46%)
Adenomyepithelioma	4(1,34%)
Papilloma	3 (1,01 %)
Other	17 (5,70 %)

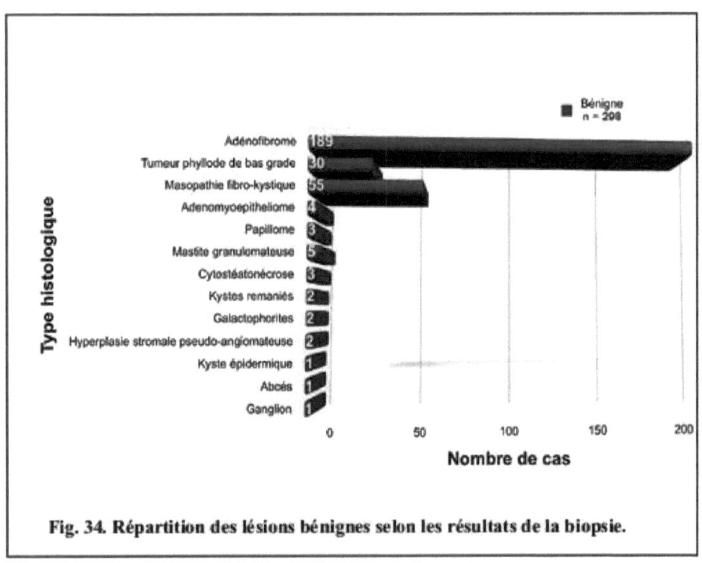

Fig. 34. Répartition des lésions bénignes selon les résultats de la biopsie.

Fig. 34. Distribution of benign lesions according to biopsy results.

4.1.2. Malignant lesions

4.1.2.1. Histological types

Pathological analysis of the malignant lesions revealed two ductal carcinomas in situ (2.60%) and 75 infiltrating carcinomas (97.40%) (table 53).

Among the infiltrating carcinomas, we found 55 NST carcinomas at biopsy, i.e. 73.33% of infiltrating carcinomas, nine lobular carcinomas, four mixed carcinomas, two micro-papillary carcinomas, one papillary intracystic carcinoma, one cribriform carcinoma, one colloid carcinoma, one apocrine carcinoma and one neuroendocrine carcinoma (fig. 35).

Table 53. Distribution of malignant masses according to biopsy results.				
Mass	**Malignant n = 77**			
Histological type	**NST**	**Lobular**	**Mixed**	**Other**
Carcinoma in situ	2 (100 %)	0	0	0
Invasive carcinoma	55 (73,33 %)	9 (12,02 %)	4 (5,33 %)	7 (9,33 %)

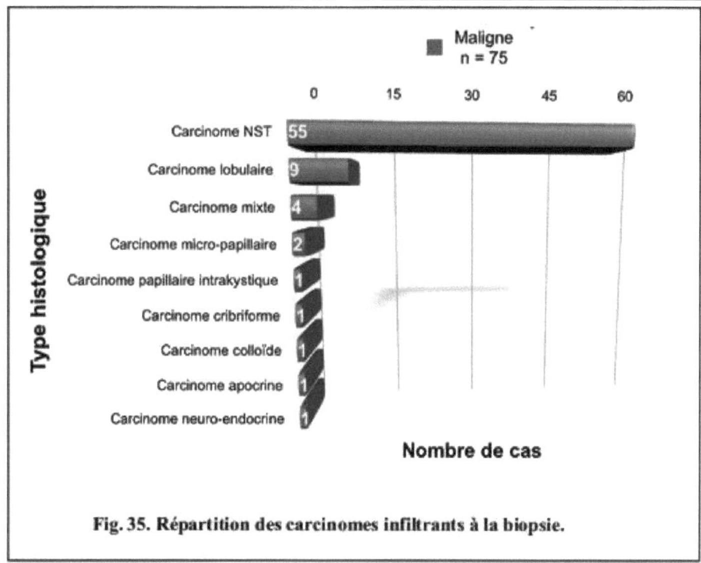

Fig. 35. Distribution of infiltrating carcinomas at biopsy.

4.1.2.2. Histo-pronostic grade

Table 54 summarises the distribution of malignant lesions according to histological grade and shows that the majority of infiltrating carcinomas were grade II (76%).

Table 54. Histological grade distribution of infiltrating carcinomas at biopsy.	
Mass	**Malignant n = 75**
Histo-pronostic grade	
I	7 (9,33 %)
II	57 (76,00 %)
III	11 (14,67%)

4.1.2.3. Hormone receptors

Invasive carcinomas frequently expressed mstrogen and progesterone receptors, 85.33% and 78.67% respectively (table 55).

Table 55. Distribution according to hormone receptor expression of infiltrating carcinomas at biopsy.	
Mass	**Malignant n = 75**
Estrogen receptor	
Positive	64 (85,33 %)
Negative	11 (14,67%)
Progesterone receptor	
Positive	59 (78,67 %)
Negative	16(21,33%)

4.1.2.4. HER2 status

As shown in Table 56, infiltrating carcinomas rarely overexpressed HER2 growth factors (10.67%).

Table 56. Distribution according to HER2 overexpression of invasive carcinomas at biopsy.	
Mass	**Malignant n = 75**
HER2 status	
Positive	8 (10,67%)
Negative	67 (89,33%)

4.1.2.5. Proliferation index

The majority of invasive carcinomas in our series (81.33%) had a high proliferation index and only 18.67% had a low proliferation index (table 57).

Table 57. Distribution according to proliferation index of infiltrating carcinomas at biopsy.	
Mass	**Malignant n = 75**
Ki 67%	
< 14	14(18,67%)
> 14	61 (81,33 %)

4.1.2.6. Molecular classification

The 75 invasive carcinomas were classified according to molecular classification as luminal A in 12 cases (16%), luminal B in 52 cases (69.33%), HER2 in 4 cases (5.33%) and triple negative in 7 cases (9.33%) (Table 58).

We note that the luminal type B was more frequently found.

Table 58. Molecular classification of invasive carcinomas at biopsy.	
Mass	**Malignant n = 75**
Molecular classification	
Luminal A	12 (16,00%)
Luminal B	52 (69,33%)
HER2	4 (5,33%)

Triple negative	7 (9,33%)

4.2. Results of the study of the surgical specimen

Thirty-four patients with malignant lesions, i.e. 47.22% (37 masses out of 77 [48.05%]), underwent additional surgery, including four lumpectomies, 6 lumpectomies with curage and 24 mastectomies with curage.

4.2.1. Size

The mean size of the 37 masses on the surgical specimen was 24.11 + 15.89 mm, with extremes ranging from 5 mm to 90 mm.

The distribution of malignant masses according to size on the operative specimens, by size range of 0 mm, shows a peak in the 11-20 mm range (fig. 36).

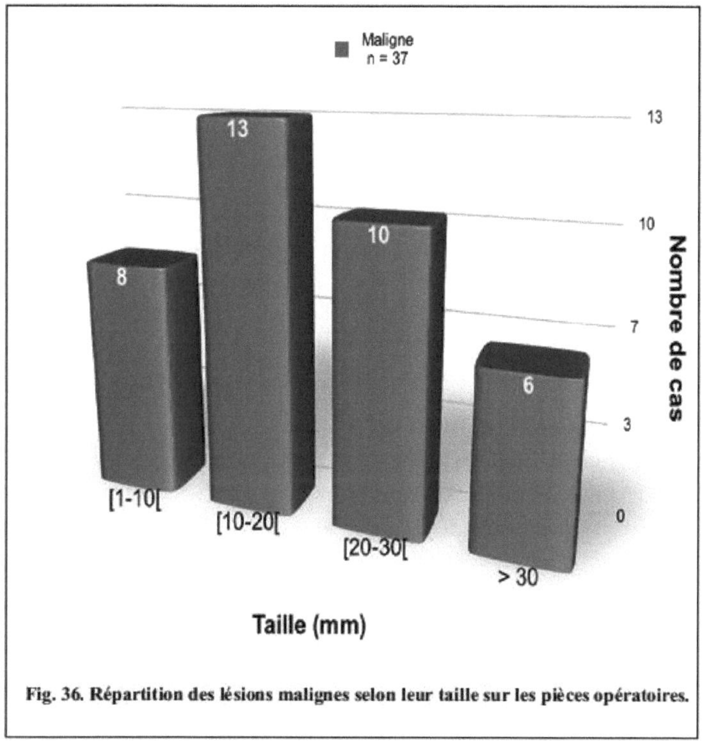

Fig. 36. Répartition des lésions malignes selon leur taille sur les pièces opératoires.

Fig. 36. Distribution of malignant lesions according to size on surgical specimens.

4.2.2. Histological type

Anatomopathological examination of the surgical specimens revealed 36 infiltrating carcinomas (97.30%) and one case of ductal carcinoma in situ (2.70%) (table 59).

Among the invasive carcinomas, we found 26 NST carcinomas, i.e. 72.22% of invasive carcinomas, three lobular carcinomas, three mixed carcinomas, one micro-papillary carcinoma, one papillary intra-cystic carcinoma, one colloid carcinoma and one apocrine carcinoma (fig.37).

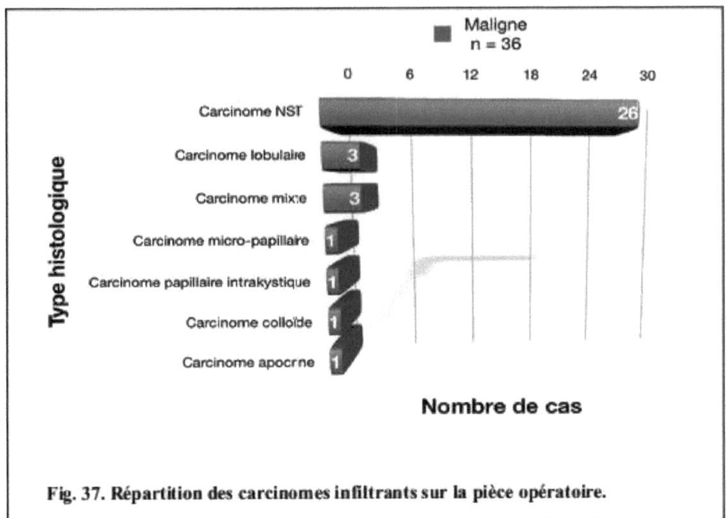

Fig. 37. Répartition des carcinomes infiltrants sur la pièce opératoire.

Fig. 37. Distribution of infiltrating carcinomas on the surgical specimen.

Table 59. Distribution of malignant lesions according to surgical findings.				
Mass	**Malignant n = 37**			
Histological type	**NST**	**Lobular**	**Mixed**	**Other**
Carcinoma in situ	**1 (100%)**	0	0	**0**
Invasive carcinoma	26 (72,22%)	3 (8,33%)	3 (8,33%)	3 (11,11%)

4.2.3. Histo-pronostic grade

Of the 36 infiltrating malignant lesions, 26 were grade II (72.22%), 2 grade I (5.56%) and 8 grade III (22.22%) (table 60).

Table 60. Histological grade distribution of invasive carcinomas in operated patients.	
Mass	**Malignant η = 36**
Histo-pronostic grade	
I	2 (5,56 %)
II	26 (72,22 %)
III	8 (22,22%)

4.2.4. Hormone receptors

In the 36 infiltrating carcinomas analysed on the surgical specimen, mstrogen and progesterone receptors were frequently expressed, respectively 86.11% and 77.78% (table 61).

Table 61. Distribution according to hormone receptor expression of infiltrating carcinomas on the surgical specimen.	
Mass	**Malignant n = 36**

Estrogen receptor	
Positive	31 (86,11%)
Negative	5 (13,89%)
Progesterone receptor	
Positive	28 (77,78%)
Negative	8 (22,22%)

4.2.5. HER2 status

As shown in Table 62, infiltrating carcinomas rarely overexpressed HER2 growth factors (13.89%).

Table 62. Distribution of infiltrating carcinomas on the surgical specimen according to HER2 overexpression.

Mass	**Malignant n = 36**
HER2 status	
Positive	5 (13,89%)
Negative	31(86,11%)

4.2.6. Proliferation index

The majority of invasive carcinomas (83.33%) had a high proliferation index and only 16.67% had a low proliferation index (table 63).

Table 63. Distribution of infiltrating carcinomas on the surgical specimen according to the proliferation index.

Mass	**Malignant n = 36**
Ki 67	
< 14	6(16,67%)
> 14	30 (83,33 %)

4.2.7. Molecular classification

The 36 invasive carcinomas were classified according to molecular classification as luminal A in 3 cases (8.33%), luminal B in 29 cases (80.56%), HER2 in 3 cases (8.33%) and triple negative in one case (2.78%) (Table 64).

Table 64. Molecular classification of invasive carcinomas at surgery.

Mass	**Malignant η = 36**
Molecular classification	
Luminal A	3 (8,33%)
Luminal B	29 (80,56%)
HER2	3 (8,3 %)
Triple negative	1 (2,78%)

4.2.8. Vascular emboli

Vascular emboli were found in only three cases (8.33%) and the lesions were of the infiltrating ductal type (table 65).

Table 65. Distribution of invasive carcinomas according to vascular invasion.	
Mass	**Malignant n = 36**
Vascular emboli	
Presence	3 (8,33%)
Absence	33 (91,67%)

4.2.9. Necrosis

Anatomopathological analysis revealed 4 cases of intra-tumoral necrosis out of 36 infiltrating carcinomas. Most of the infiltrating carcinomas did not show necrosis (88.89%) (table 66).

Table 66. Distribution of infiltrating carcinomas according to the presence of necrosis.	
Mass	**Malignant n = 36**
Necrosis	
Presence	4(11,11 %)
Absence	32(88,89 %)

4.2.10. Mucine

Only one case showed mucin in the operative specimens. The lesion was of the colloid carcinoma type (table 67).

Table 67. Distribution of infiltrating carcinomas according to the presence of mucin.	
Mass	**Malignant n = 36**
Mucine	
Presence	1 (2,78 %)
Absence	35 (97,22 %)

4.2.11. Fibrosis

As shown in Table 68, most of the invasive carcinomas in our series showed moderate (55.56%) and rarely extensive (11.11%) peri-tumoral fibrosis.

Table 68. Distribution according to the abundance of peritumoral fibrosis in infiltrating carcinomas.	
Mass	**Malignant η = 36**
Abundance of fibrosis	
A little bewildering	12 (33,33%)
Weighted average	20 (55,56%)
Trés ahondante	4(11,11%)

4.2.12. Ganglion

After analysis of the axillary lymph nodes, 19 patients (55.88%) had non-infiltrated lymph nodes and 15 patients (44.12%) had infiltrated lymph nodes (table 69).

Table 69. Distribution of invasive carcinomas according to lymph node

infiltration.	
Patient	**Malignant n = 34**
Node infiltration	
Negative	19 (55,88%)
Positive	15 (44,12%)

5. Correlations of elastography parameters

5.2. Threshold values - benign versus malignant

5.1.1. Elasticity score

The best threshold value of the elasticity score for differentiating between benign and malignant masses was between score 3 and 4 (Youden Index [YI] = 0.873) with an area under the curve (AUC) of 0.972, a sensitivity of 89.6% and a specificity of 97.7% (fig. 38).

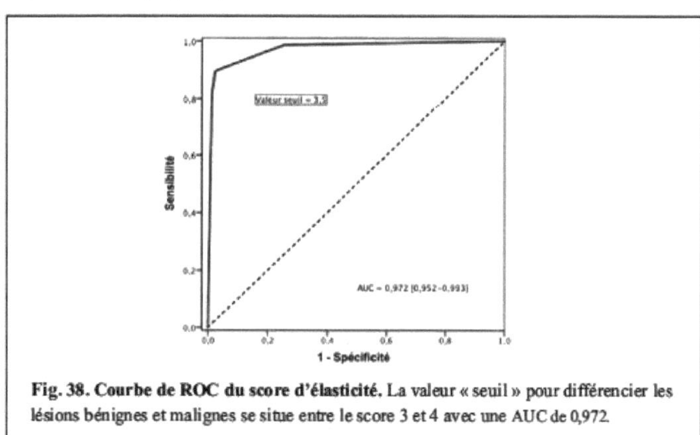

Fig. 38. Courbe de ROC du score d'élasticité. La valeur « seuil » pour différencier les lésions bénignes et malignes se situe entre le score 3 et 4 avec une AUC de 0,972.

Fig. 38. ROC curve for the elasticity score. The "threshold" value for differentiating benign and malignant lesions lies between score 3 and 4 with an AUC of 0.972.

5.1.2. Elasticity ratio

The best threshold values for the fat-to-lesion ratio (FLR) and gland-to-lesion ratio (GLR) were 3.67 (IY = 0.881) and 1.87 (IY = 0.531) respectively.

The sensitivity, specificity and AUC of the FLR were, respectively, 96.1%, 93.3% and 0.990, CI [0.981-0.999]. The corresponding GLR values were 72%, 81.1% and 0.820, CI [0.740-0.900] respectively.

In terms of diagnostic performance (sensitivity, specificity and AUC), FLR was significantly superior to GLR ($p < 0.0001$) (fig. 39).

To this end, we chose the FLR as the quantitative elastography parameter.

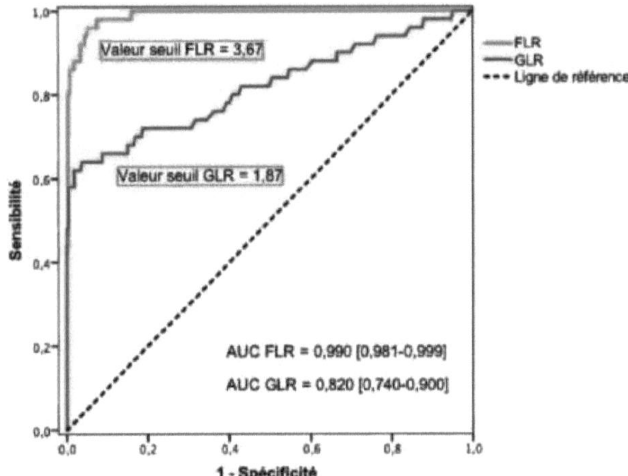

Fig. 39. ROC curve for the elasticity ratio. FLR threshold value of 3.67 with an AUC of 0.990. GLR threshold value of 1.87 with an AUC of 0.820.

5.1.3. Size ratio

With a best threshold value calculated at 1.045 (Youden Index [YI] = 0.85), the size ratio shows a sensitivity of 87%, a specificity of 80% and an area under the curve (AUC) of 0.951 (fig. 40).

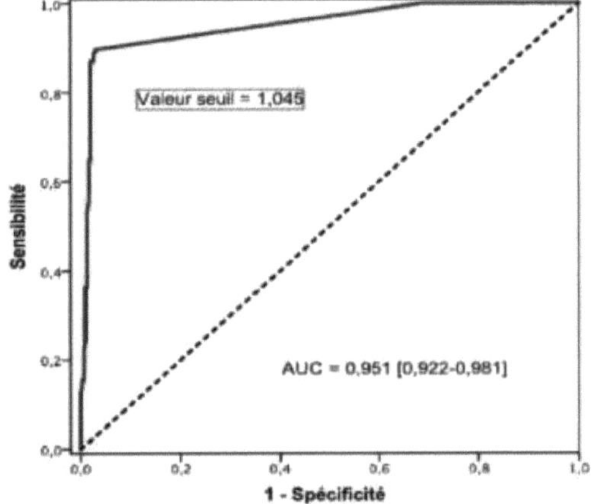

Fig. 40. ROC curve of the size ratio. Threshold value for differentiating benign and malignant lesions is 1.045 with an AUC of 0.972.

5.2. Correlations between population data and elastographic parameters

5.2.1. Age

We compared concordant elastographic results (scores 1, 2, 3 and elasticity ratio values below the 3.67 threshold were found in benign lesions and scores 4, 5 and elasticity ratio values greater than or equal to the 3,67 are found in malignant lesions) and discordant results (benign lesions are scored 4, 5 and had elasticity ratio values greater than or equal to the threshold 3.67 and malignant lesions are scored 1, 2, 3 and had elasticity ratio values less than the threshold 3.67).

We found no significant difference between the concordant and discordant groups according to age (p > 0.05) (table 70).

Table 70. Correlations between elastographic parameters and patient age.

Weights	**Benign η = 298**			**Malignant η = 77**		
Elasticity score	**Matching images (1,2,3)**	**Discordant images (4, 5)**	*P*	**Concordant images (4, 5)**	**Discordant images (1,2,3)**	*p*
Age (years)	**η (%)**	**η (%)**	0,22	**η (%)**	**η (%)**	0,60
<40	130 (44,7 %)	1 (14,3 %)		5 (7,2 %)	1 (12,5 %)	
>40	161 (55,3 %)	6 (85,7 %)		64 (92,8 %)	7 (87,5 %)	
Elasticity ratio	**Concordant results <3.67**	**Discordant results >3.67**	*P*	**Concordant results >3.67**	**Discordant results <3.67**	*P*
Age (years)	**η (%)**	**η (%)**	0,81	**η (%)**	**η (%)**	0,61
<40	123 (44,2%)	8 (40,0 %)		6(8,1 %)	**0**	
>40	155 (55,8 %)	12 (60,0 %)		68 (91,9%)	3 (100 %)	

5.2.2. Body mass index (BMI)

According to the results in Table 71, there was no significant difference between the concordant and discordant groups in the elastographic results according to body mass index (p > 0.05).

Table 71. Correlations between elastographic results and patient BMI.

Weights	Benign η = 298			Malignant η =77		
Elasticity score	Matching images (1, 2, 3)	Discordant images (4, 5)	*P*	Concordant images (4, 5)	Discordant images (1, 2, 3)	*P*
BMI	η (%)	η (%)	0,098	η (%)	η (%)	0,051
Leanness< 18.5	17 (5,8 %)	1 (14,3 %)		0	0	
Normal [18.5-25[	122 (41,9 %)	0		13 (18,8 %)	4 (50,0 %)	
Overweight[25-30[	101 (34,7 %)	3 (42,9 %)		32 (46,4 %)	4 (50,0 %)	
Obesity >30	51 (17,5 %)	3 (42,9 %)		24 (34,8 %)	0	
Elasticity ratio	Concordant results <3.67	Discordant results >3.67	*P*	Concordant results >3.67	Discordant results <3.67	*P*
BMI	η (%)	η (%)	0,56	η (%)	η (%)	0,14
Leanness< 18.5	17 (6,0 %)	1 (5,0 %)		0	0	
Normal [18.5-25[	115(41,4%)	7 (35,0 %)		15 (20,3 %)	2 (66,7 %)	
Overweight[25-30[	98 (35,3 %)	6 (30,0 %)		35 (47,3 %)	1 (33,3 %)	
Obesity >30	48 (17,3 %)	6 (30,0 %)		24 (32,4 %)	0	

5.3. Correlations of palpable masses and elastographic parameters

In table 72, score 5 was more frequently found in palpable masses than in non-palpable masses (33.58% vs 8.82%,j9 < *0.0001)*.

Mean lesion hardness was significantly higher for palpable lesions than for non-palpable lesions (15.11 + 31.79 vs 4.49 + 11.53,ρ< *0.0001).*
86.6% of non-palpable masses had an elasticity ratio below the defined threshold (FLR <3.67).
The mean size ratio was higher in palpable masses 1.09 + 0.17 than in non-palpable masses 1.04 + 0.*15,p< 0.0001.*

Table 72. Correlations between palpable masses and elastographic parameters.

Mass	**Palpable η = 137**	**Not palpable η = 238**	*ρ*
Elastography parameters			
Colorimetric score	**η (%)**	**η (%)**	
1	2(1,46%)	8 (3,36 %)	**< 0,0001**
2	51 (37,23 %)	162 (68,07 %)	
3	34 (24,82 %)	42 (17,65 %)	
4	4 (2,92 %)	5 (2,10 %)	
5	46 (33,58 %)	21 (8,82 %)	
Elasticity ratio (mean + standard deviation)	15,11 ±31,79	4,49 ± 11,53	**< 0,0001**
Size ratio (mean + standard deviation)	1,09 ±0,17	1,04 ±0,15	**0,004**

5.4. Correlation of mammographic and elastographic parameters

5.4.1. Breast density

Among the malignant lesions, patients with extremely dense breasts (density d) made up 25% of the group of discordant images, which is much more than the 2.9% in the concordant group *(p = 0.007).*
Among the benign lesions, patients with completely fatty breasts (density a) made up 57.1% of the group of discordant images, which is significantly higher than the 10.7% of concordant group *(p = 0.0002).*
The elasticity ratio showed no difference between the concordant and discordant groups *(ρ = 0.28*) (table 73).

Table 73. Correlations between mammographic breast density and elastography results.

Weights	**Benign n = 204**			**Malignant η =77**		
Elasticity score	**Matching images (1,2,3)**	**Discordant images (4, 5)**	*ρ*	**Concordant images (4, 5)**	**Discordant images (1,2,3)**	*ρ*
Breast density	**η (%)**	**η (%)**	**0,001**	**η (%)**	**η (%)**	**0,02**
a	21 (10,7 %)	4(57,1 %)		25 (36,2 %)	2 (25,0 %)	
b	94 (47,7 %)	2 (28,6 %)		29 (42 %)	1 (12,5 %)	
c	71 (36,0 %)	0		13 (18,8 %)	3 (37,5 %)	
d	11 (5,6%)	1 (14,3 %)		2 (2,9 %)	2 (25,0 %)	
Elasticity	**Concordant**	**Discordant**	*P*	**Concordant**	**Discordant**	*P*

ratio	results <3.67	results >3.67		results >3.67	results <3.67	
Breast density	η (%)	η (%)	0,21	η (%)	η (%)	0,28
a	21 (11,2%)	4 (25,0 %)		25 (34,2 %)	2 (75,0 %)	
b	91 (48,7%)	5 (31,3 %)		30(41,1 %)	**0**	
c	66 (35,1 %)	5 (31,3 %)		14 (19,2 %)	1 (25,0 %)	
d	10 (5,3 %)	2 (12,5 %)		4 (5,5 %)	**0**	

5.4.2. Visible masses

As shown in table 74, scores 4 and 5 were more often found in lesions visible on mammography than in lesions not visible (42.1% vs 6%, $p < 0.0001$). Conversely, masses not visible on mammography were often scored 1, 2 and 3 (94.0% vs 57.9%,j9 < *0.0001).*

The mean lesion hardness was higher for lesions visible on mammography than for those hidden by mammography (15.88 + 31.24 vs 2.98 + 5.10,_p < *0.0001*) (fig. 41).

88.9% of lesions hidden on mammography had an elasticity ratio below the defined threshold of 3.67.

Table 74. Correlations between masses visible on mammography and elastographic parameters.			
Mass	**Visible η = 164**	**Not visible η = 120**	*P*
Elastography parameters			
Colorimetric score			**< 0,0001**
1	1 (0,6 %)	6(5,1 %)	
2	58 (35,4 %)	78 (66,7 %)	
3	36 (22,0 %)	26 (22,2 %)	
4	7 (4,3 %)	2(1,7%)	
5	62 (37,8 %)	5 (4,3 %)	
Elasticity ratio (mean + standard deviation)	15,90 ±31,24	2,98 ±5,10	**< 0,0001**
Size ratio (mean + standard deviation)	1,10 ±0,20	1 ± 0,069	**< 0,0001**

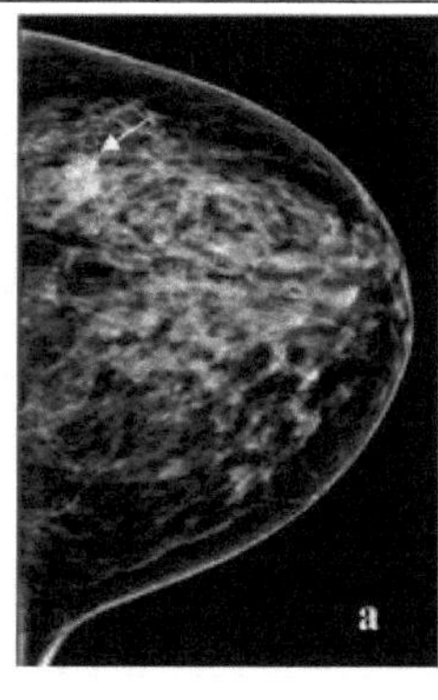

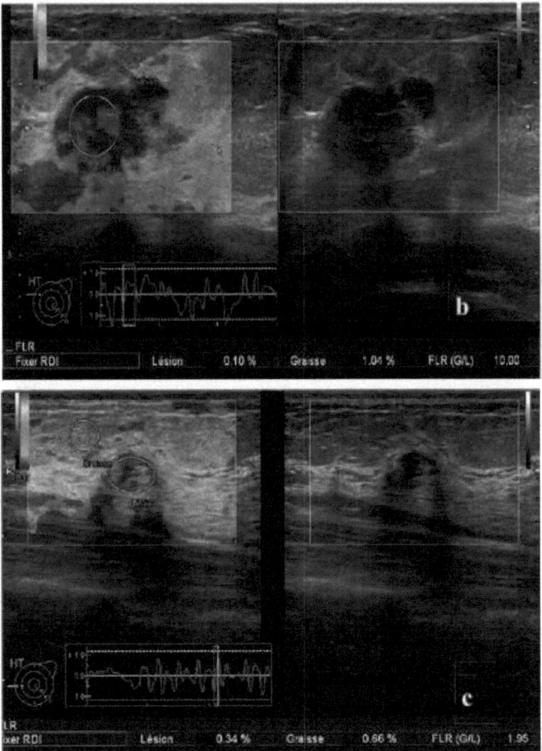

Fig. 41: Visibility of masses on mammography. A 43-year-old woman with two breast lumps. (a) Mammogram. A visible mass, oval in shape, with irregular contours, hyperdense (arrow). (b) Elastography. The mass visible on mammography, with an elasticity score of 5 and an elasticity ratio calculated at 10. Invasive carcinoma NST. (c) The mass not visible on mommography, with an elasticity score of 2 and a calculated elasticity ratio of 1.95. Fibroadenoma.

5.5. Correlation of ultrasound and elastographic parameters

5.5.1. Mass size

The mean major axis of lesions with an elasticity score above the determined threshold (score 4 and 5) was significantly greater than that of lesions with an elasticity score below the threshold (score 1, 2 and 3) (22.45 + 11.13 vs 18.28 + 11.01,p = 0.003) (table 75).

The mean major axis of the masses increased as the elasticity score increased. The Spearman correlation coefficient between the elasticity score and the mean major axis of the lesions was significant, with a value of 0.23 ($p < 0.0001$) (table 76) (fig. 42).

Similarly, lesions with elasticity and size ratios above the threshold were larger than those with ratios below the threshold (table 75).

Table 75. Correlations between average mass size and elastography parameters.			
Average mass size (mm)	**Above threshold value (mean + standard deviation)**	**Below threshold value (mean + standard deviation)**	*P*
Elastography parameters			
Elasticity score	22,45 ± 11,13	18,28 ± 11,01	**0,003**
Elasticity ratio	22,51 ±11,27	17,99 ± 10,89	**0,001**
Size ratio	23,38 ± 12,04	18,09 ± 10,69	< **0,0001**

Table 76. Correlations between mean mass size and colorimetric score.				
Mass	**n = 375**	**Size in mm** **(mean + standard deviation)**	*rho*	*P*
Elastography parameters				
Elasticity score			**0,23**	**0,003**
1	10	11,89 ±4,41		
2	213	17,73 ±9,81		
3	76	20,63 ± 13,98		
4	**9**	19,92 ±8,53		
5	**67**	22,79 ± 11,45		

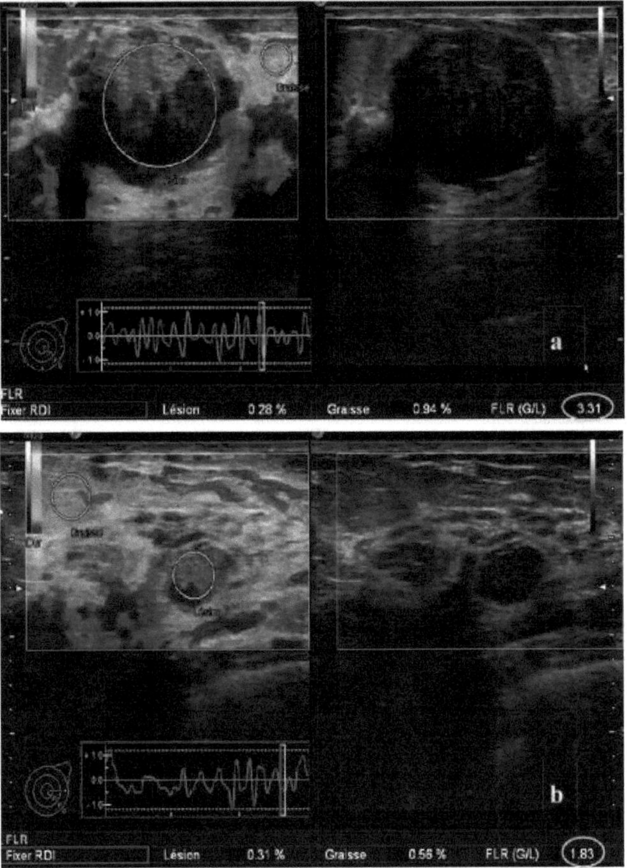

Fig. 42: Two lesions of juvenile fibroadenoma in a 22-year-old female patient. Elastographic image: (a) Large mass 27.7 mm long, scored 3 on elastography, calculated elasticity ratio 3.31. (b) 10.6 mm long axis mass, scored 2 on elastography, calculated elasticity ratio 1.83.

Malignant discordant elastographic colour images were larger on average than concordant elastographic images (32.80 + 12.78 versus 23.49 + 11.08,^ = *0.04*). However, the benign discordant elastographic images were relatively smaller in size than the concordant elastographic images (12.10 + 4.54 versus 17.87 + 10.71, *p = 0.002*) (figs. 43 and 44).

The elasticity and size ratios showed no difference between the concordant and discordant groups (p > 0.05) (table 77).

Table 77. Correlations between elastography results and mass size.						
Weights	**Benign n = 298**			**Malignant n =77**		
Size (mm) **(average + standard deviation)**	**Consistent results**	**Discordant results**	*P*	**Consistent results**	**Discordant results**	*P*

Elastography parameters						
Elasticity score	17,87 + 10,71	12,10 + 4,54	**0,002**	23,49+ 11,08	32,80+ 12,78	**0,04**
Elasticity ratio	17,86+10,86	16,12 + 6,80	0,29	24,24+ 11,65	29,93 + 7,34	0,2
Size ratio	17,74+10,34	22,15 ±21,91	0,62	23,49 ± 11,03	30,96+ 13,28	**0,09**

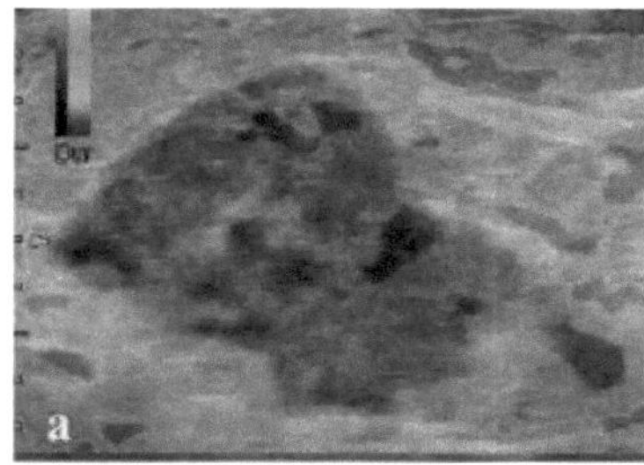

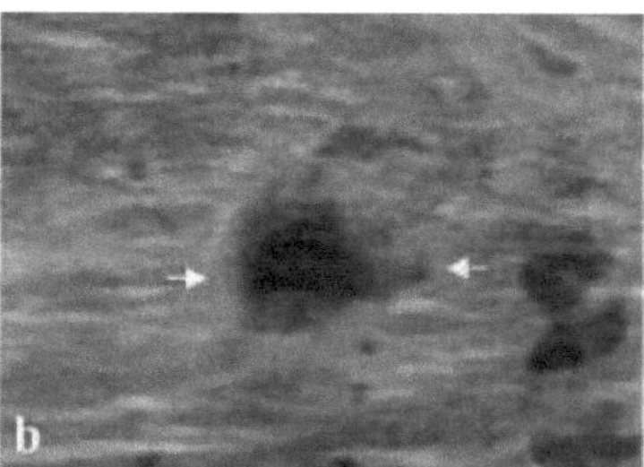

Fig. 43: NST infiltrating carcinoma lesions. Elastographic image: (a) Large mass 26 mm long, scored 2; (b) mass 6.2 mm long, scored 5 (arrows).

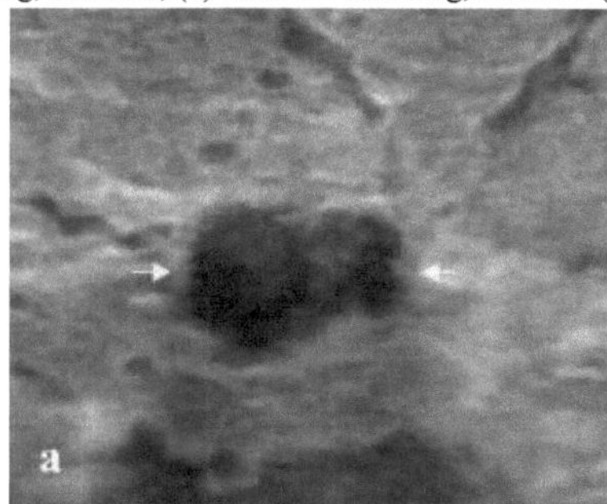

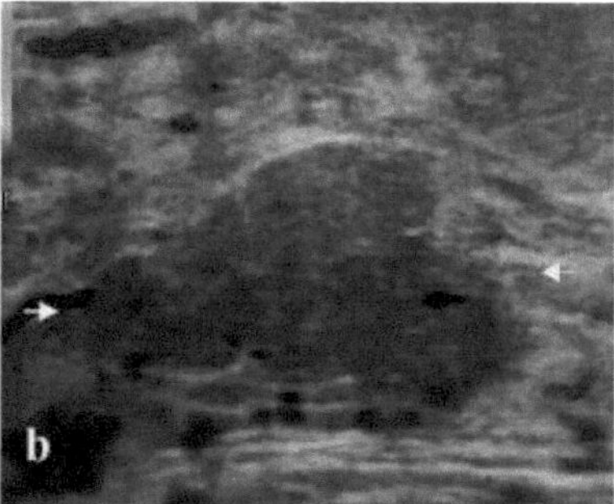

Fig. 44: Fibroadenoma lesions. Elastographic image: (a) 10.5 mm long-axis mass, scored 4 (arrows). (b) Large mass 31.4 mm long, scored 1 (arrows).

5.5.2. Distance to nipple

As shown in Table 78, there was no significant difference between the mean distance of the masses from the nipple and the elastographic results in the concordant and discordant groups ($p > 0.05$).

Table 78. Correlations between distance from the nipple and elastographic results.

Weights	**Benign η = 298**			**Malignant η =77**		
Nipple distance (mm) (average + standard deviation)	**Concordant results**	**Discordant results**	*P*	**Concordant results**	**Discordant results**	*P*
Elastography parameters						
Elasticity score	41,52 + 21,83	40,64 + 25,79	0,92	44,66 + 27,48	49,86 + 29,36	0,63
Elasticity ratio	41,81+21,51	37,13 +26,77	0,44	44,27 + 27,02	68,13 + 31,04	0,19

5.5.3. Distance to the pean

Analysis of Table 79 revealed no significant difference between the mean distance of the lesions from the skin and the elastographic results of the concordant and discordant groups (p > 0.05).

Table 79. Correlations between distance from the pean and elastographic results.						
Weights	**Benign n = 298**			**Malignant n =77**		
Distance from skin (mm) (mean + standard deviation)	**Concordant results**	**Discordant results**	*P*	**Concordant results**	**Discordant results**	*P*
Elastography parameters						
Elasticity score	8,36 ±5,36	7,18 ± 8,18	0,07	7,46 ± 4,73	5,69 ±3,57	0,2
Elasticity ratio	8,54 ±5,46	6,36 ±4,13	0,06	7,32 ±4,70	6,13 ±2,80	0,5

5.5.4. Breast thickness

As shown in Table 80, there was no significant difference between mean breast thickness and elastographic results in the concordant and discordant groups (p > 0.05).

Table 80. Correlations between breast thickness and elastography results.						
Weights	**Benign n = 298**		*P*	**Malignant η =77**		*P*
Breast thickness (mm) (mean + standard deviation)	**Concordant results**	**Discordant results**		**Concordant results**	**Discordant results**	
Elastography parameters						
Elasticity score	35,07± 14,67	56,57 + 34,16	0,1	38,84+ 13,58	30,97 + 7,42	0,1
Elasticity ratio	34,82+ 14,52	45,98 + 25,04	0,06	38,26+ 13,47	35,00 + 3,40	0,19

5.5.5. Calcifications

In Table 81, we noted no significant difference between the concordant and discordant elastographic results related to the presence or absence of calcifications in the mass *(p>0.05)* (figs. 45 and 46).

Table 81. Correlations between elastographic results and the presence of calcifications.						
Weights	**Benign η = 298**		*P*	**Malignant η = 77**		*P*
Elasticity score	**Matching images (1, 2, 3)**	**Discordant images (4, 5)**		**Concordant images (4, 5)**	**Discordant images (1, 2, 3)**	
Calcifications			0,35			0,22
Present	39(13,4%)	2 (28,6 %)		38 (55,1 %)	2 (25,0 %)	
Absent	252 (86,6 %)	5(71,4%)		31 (44,9 %)	6 (75,0 %)	
Elasticity ratio	**Concordant results <3.67**	**Discordant results >3.67**		**Concordant results >3.67**	**Discordant results <3.67**	
Calcifications			0,61			0,94
Present	37 (13,3 %)	4 (20,0 %)		39 (52,7 %)	1 (33,3 %)	
Absent	241 (86,7 %)	16(80,0%)		35 (47,3 %)	2 (66,7 %)	

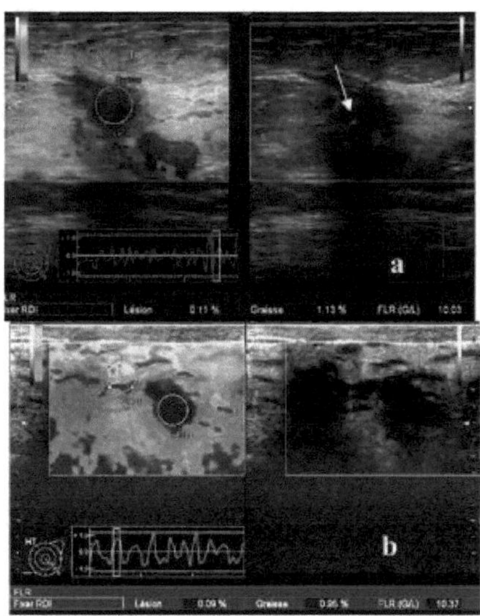

Fig. 45: Intra-lesional calcifications and elastography. (a) Malignant mass, showing calcifications on ultrasound mode B (arrow), with an elasticity ratio of 10.03 on elastography. Carcinoma inflltrant type NST. (b) Malignant mass, without calcifications within it, with elasticity ratio of 10.37 on elastography. NST infllrant carcinoma.

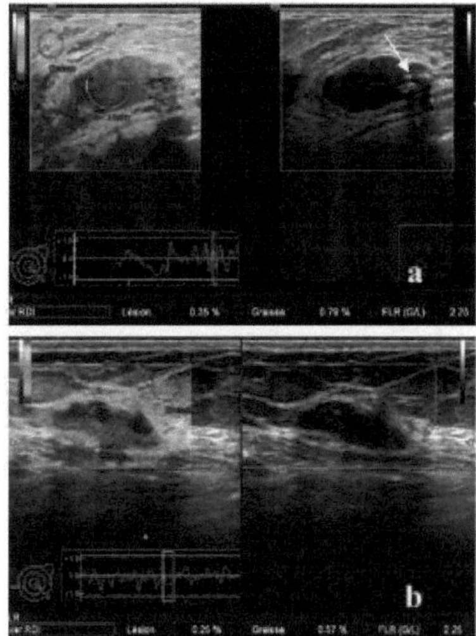

Fig. 46: Intra-lesional calcifications and elastography.
(a) Benign mass, showing calcifications on ultrasound mode B (arrow), scored 2 and with an elasticity ratio of 2.23 on elastography. Fibroadenoma. (b) Benign mass, without calcifications within it, scored 2 and with an elasticity ratio of 2.25 on elastography. Fibroadenoma.

5.5.6. Vascularisation

Analysis of table 82 shows no significant difference between the concordant and discordant elastographic results related to the presence or absence of vascularisation in the lesions *(p>0, 05)* (figs. 47 and 48).

Table 82. Correlations of elastographic results and vascularisation using colour Doppler.

Weights	Benign n = 298		*P*	Malignant n = 77		*P*
Elasticity score	Matching images (1, 2, 3)	Discordant images (4, 5)		Concordant images (4, 5)	Discordant images (1, 2, 3)	
Vascularisation			0,36			0,56
Present	228 (78,4 %)	7(100%)		66 (95,7 %)	8(100%)	
Absent	63 (21,6 %)	0		3 (4,3 %)	0	
Elasticity ratio	Concordant results < 3.67	Discordant results >3.67		Concordant results >3.67	Discordant results <3.67	
Vascularisation			0,35			0,72
Present	217 (78,1%)	18(90,0%)		71 (95,9 %)	3 (100%)	
Absent	61(21,9 %)	2(10,0%)		3 (4,1 %)	0	

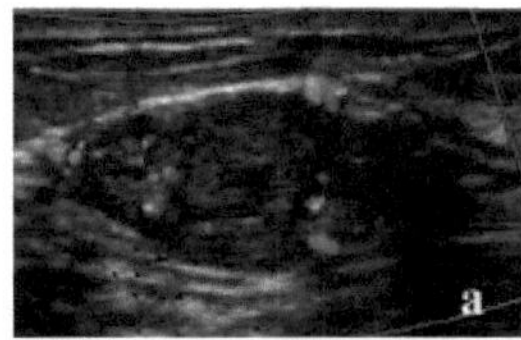

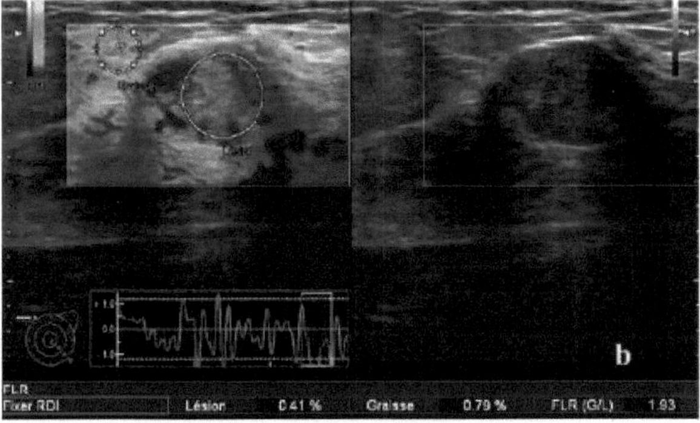

Fig. 47: Intra-lesional vascularisation and elastography. (a) Mass with central and peripheral vascularisation on colour Doppler. (b) On elastography, the mass scored 2 and 1.93 elasticity ratio. Fibroadenoma.

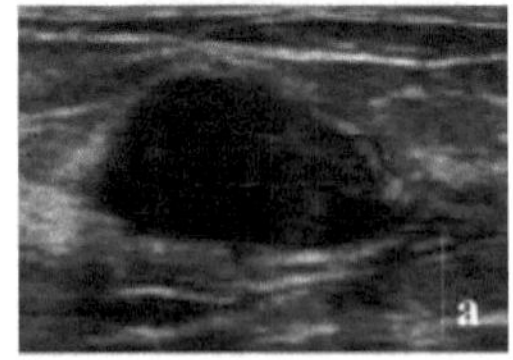

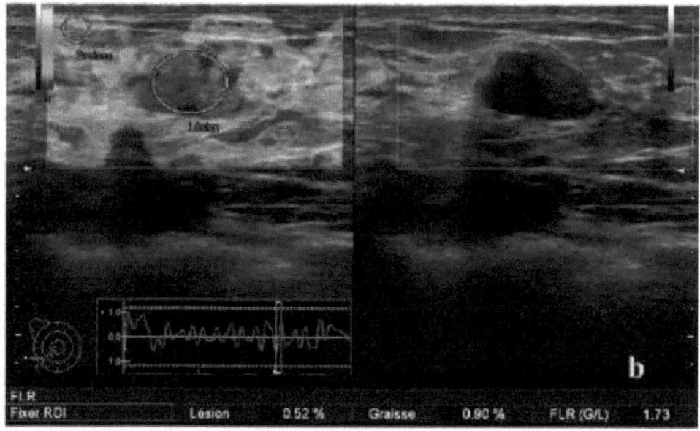

Fig. 48: Intra-lesional vascularisation and elastography. (a) Vascular pen mass on colour Doppler. (b) On elastography, the mass scored 2 and 1.73 elasticity ratio. Fibroadenoma.

5.5.7. BI-RADS category

The distribution of elasticity parameters and the BI-RADS classification are shown in table 83.

76 masses classified as BI-RADS 3 were scored 1, 2 and 3 (fig.49).

Of the lesions classified as BI-RADS 5, 54 lesions (98.2%) were scored 4 or 5 (fig. 50). One BI-RADS 5 lesion (1.8%) was graded 3, the histological result revealing a cytosteatonecrosis lesion.

For lesions classified as BI-RADS 4, elasticity scores ranged from 1 to 5 (figs. 51 and 52).

A total of 222 masses (90.98%) were graded 1, 2 or 3 and 22 lesions were graded 4 or 5.

Correlations between elastography parameters (elasticity and size ratio) and BI-RADS categories are reported in Table 84, which shows that elasticity and size ratio values increased significantly with BI-RADS categories *(p < 0.0001).*

Table 83. Distribution of elasticity score and BI-RADS categories.

Category BI-RADS	**Histology (n = 375)**	**Elasticity score**					***P***
		1	**2**	3	4	**5**	**< 0,0001**
3	Benin (76)	4 (5,2 %)	54 (71,1%)	18(23,7%)	0	0	
	Malin (0)	0	0	0	0	0	
4 a	Benin (190)	5 (2,6 %)	139 (73,2 %)	42 (22,1 %)	3 (1,6%)	1 (0,5 %)	
	Malin (2)	0	1 (50,0 %)	1 (50,0 %)	0	0	
4b	Benin (7)	0	6 (85,7 %)	1 (14,3 %)	0	0	
	Malin (4)	0	0	2 (50,0 %)	2 (50,0 %)	0	
4c	Benin (23)	1 (4,3 %)	13(56,5%)	7 (30,4 %)	0	2 (8,7 %)	
	Malin (18)	0	0	4 (22,2 %)	2(11,1 %)	12(66,7%)	
5	Benin (2)	0	0	1 (50,0%)	0	1 (50,0%)	
	Malin (53)	0	0	0	2 (3,8 %)	51 (96,2%)	

Table 84. Correlations between BI-RADS categories and elastographic parameters.

Elastography parameters	Elasticity ratio (mean + standard deviation)	Size ratio (mean + standard deviation)
BI-RADS categories		

3	1,99 ± 0,93	0,98 ± 0,022
4a	2,12 + 1,31	0,99 ± 0,04
4b	2,68 ± 1,25	1,02 + 0,54
4c	7,55 ± 11,68	1,10 ± 0,20
5	40,77 ± 43,91	1,26 ± 0,22
P	< 0,0001	< 0,0001

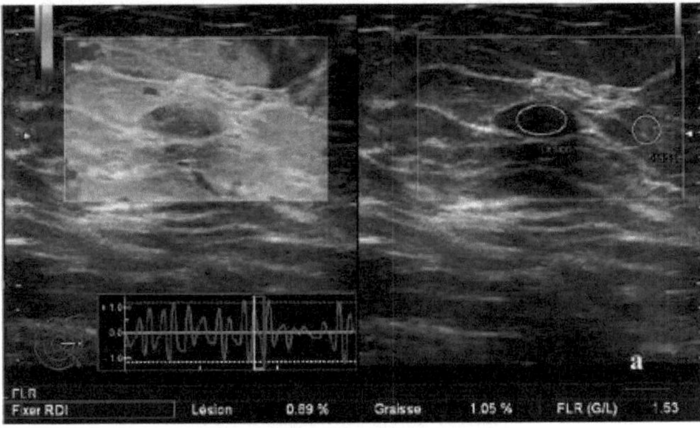

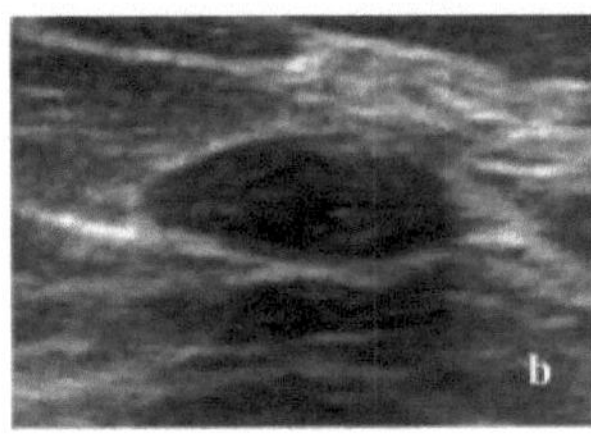

Fig. 49: Fibroadenoma in a 35-year-old woman (a) Elastographic image. Mass with an elasticity score of 2 and an elasticity ratio of 1.53. (b) Ultrasound image. Mass classified BI-RADS 3.

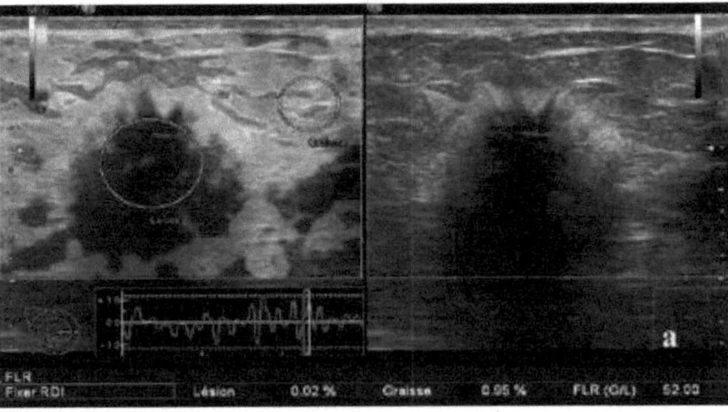

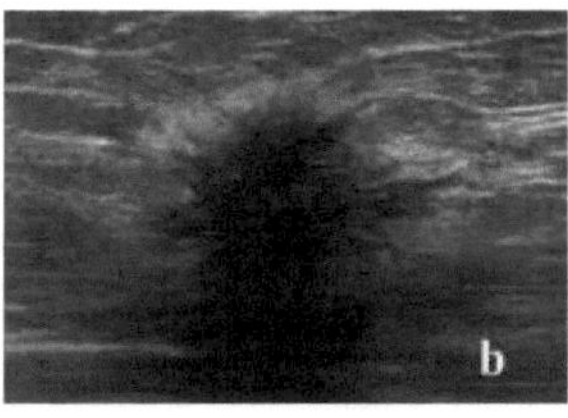

Fig. 50: Invasive NST carcinoma in a 45-year-old woman (a) Elastographic image. Mass with elasticity score 5 and elasticity ratio 52. (b) Image

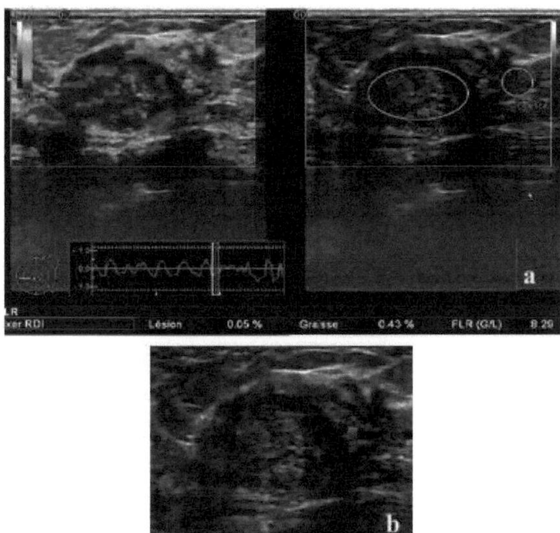

Fig. 51: Invasive colloid carcinoma in a 45-year-old woman (a) Elastographic image. Mass with an elasticity score of 4 and an elasticity ratio of 8.29. (b) Ultrasound image. Mass classified as BIRADS 4a.

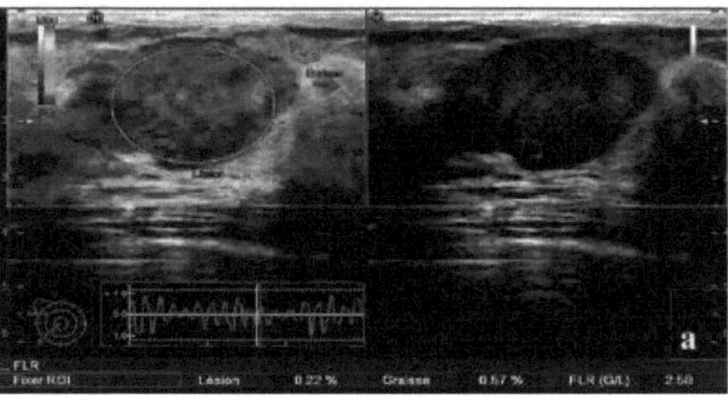

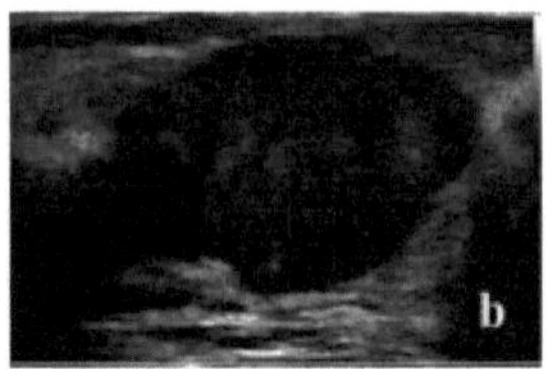

Fig. 52: Fibroadenoma in a 42-year-old woman (a) Elastographic image. Mass with an elasticity score of 3 and an elasticity ratio of 2.58. (b) Ultrasound image. Mass classified BI-RADS 4a.

5.6. Correlations between histological and elastographic results

5.6.1. Histological type

5.6.1.1. Benign lesions

Of the 298 benign masses, 219 tumours were fibro-epithelial, representing 73.49% of benign tumours, of which 189 (86.30%) were fibroadenomas and 30 (13.70%) were phyllodes. The remaining benign tumours (79 lesions or 26.51%) included fibrocystic mastopathies, adenomyo-epitheliomas, papillomas and miscellaneous lesions (figs. 53 and 54).

Benign lesions were most often scored 1, 2 and 3 in 291 cases, i.e. 97.65%, seven cases (2.35%) were scored 4 and 5, these one fibroadenoma lesion, two adenomyo-epithelioma lesions, two granulomatous mastitis lesions and two cytosteatonecrosis lesions (Table 85).

The mean value of the size ratio for adenomyo-epitheliomas, granulomatous mastitis and cytosteatonecrosis lesions was higher than for the other histological types (table 85).

The elasticity ratios for the different histological types are summarised in Table 85.

Tableau 85. Corrélation entre les types histologiques des masses bénignes et les paramètres élastographiques.

Type histologique	n =298	Paramètres d'élastographie						
		Score d'élasticité					Ratio d'élasticité (moyenne ± écart type)	Ratio de taille (moyenne ± écart type)
		1	2	3	4	5		
Fibroadénome	189 (63,4%)	4 (2,1%)	139 (73,5%)	45 (23,8%)	1 (0,5%)	0	1,97 ± 1,14	0,99 ± 0,03
Tumeur phyllode	30 (10,1%)	0	20 (66,7%)	10 (33,3%)	0	0	2,54 ± 0,83	0,99 ± 0,02
Mastopathie fibrokystique	55 (18,5%)	5 (9,1%)	42 (76,4%)	8 (14,5%)	0	0	1,86 ± 0,96	0,99 ± 0,018
Adénomyo-épithéliome	4 (1,3%)	0	2 (50,0%)	0	1 (25,0%)	1 (25,0%)	2,99 ± 2,95	1,09 ± 0,19
Papillome	3 (1%)	0	0	3 (100,0%)	0	0	2,70 ± 0,82	0,97 ± 0,05
Mastite granulomateuse	5 (1,7%)	0	2 (40,0%)	1 (20,0%)	0	2 (40,0%)	3,34 ± 2,50	1,17 ± 0,18
Cytostéatonécrose	3 (1%)	0	0	1 (33,3%)	1 (33,3%)	1 (33,3%)	3,38 ± 1,30	1,10 ± 0,17
Galactophorite	2 (0,7%)	0	2 (100,0%)	0	0	0	1,43 ± 0,60	1,00 ± 0,001
PASH	2 (0,7%)	0	2 (100,0%)	0	0	0	3,18 ± 0,59	0,99 ± 0,021
Kyste remanié	2 (0,7%)	1 (50%)	1 (50%)	0	0	0	1,87 ± 0,13	1,00 ± 0,001
Kyste épidermique	1 (0,3%)	0	0	1 (100,0%)	0	0	4,97	0,96
Abcès	1 (0,3%)	0	1 (100,0%)	0	0	0	1,26	1,15
Ganglion	1 (0,3%)	0	1 (100,0%)	0	0	0	1,23	1
P		< 0,0001					0,02	< 0,0001

Table 85. Correlation between histological types of benign masses and elastographic parameters.

Histological type	n =298	Elastography parameters						
		Elasticity score					Elasticity ratio ("novenne± standard deviation)	Size ratio ("novenne± standard deviation)
		1	2	3	4	5		
Fibroadenome	189 (63,4%)	4 (2,1%)	139 (73,5%)	45 (23,8%)	1 (0,5%)	O	1.97± 1.14	0.99± 0.03
Phyllodes tumour	30 (10,1%)	O	20 (66,7%)	IO (33.3%)	O	o	2.54± 0.83	0.99± 0.02
Fibrocystic mastopathy	55 (18,5%)	5 (9,1%)	42 (76,4%)	8 (14,5%)	O	o	1.86± 0.96	0.99± 0.018
Adenomyo-epithelioma	4 (1,3%)	O	2 (50,0%)	O	1 (25,0%)	1 (25,0%)	2.99± 2.95	1.09± 0.19
Papilloma	3 (1%)	O	O	3 (100,0%)	O	O	2.70± 0.82	0.97± 0.05
Granolomatous mastitis	5 (1,7%)	O	2 (40,0%)	1 (20,0%)	O	2 (40,0%)	3.34± 2.50	1,17 ±0,18
Oytosteatonecrosis	3 (1%)	O	O	1 (33,3%)	1 (33,3%)	1 (33,3%)	3.38± 1.30	1.10± 0.17
G>a lac top ho ri te	2 (0,7%)	0	2 (100,0%)	O	o	O	1.43± 0.60	1.00± 0.001
PASH	2 (0,7%)	o	2 (100,0%)	O	o	O	3.18± 0.59	0.99± 0.021
Cyst remanió	2 (0,7%)	1 (50%)	1 (50%)	O	o	O	1,87 ±0,13	1.00± 0.001
Epidermal cyst	1 (0,3%)	O	O	1 (100,0%)	o	O	4,97	0,96
Abscess	1 (0,3%)	O	1 (100,0%)	o	o	O	1,26	1,15
Oanglion	1 (0,3%)	o	1 (100,0%)	o	o	O	1,23	1

P			< 0,0001	0,02	< 0,0001

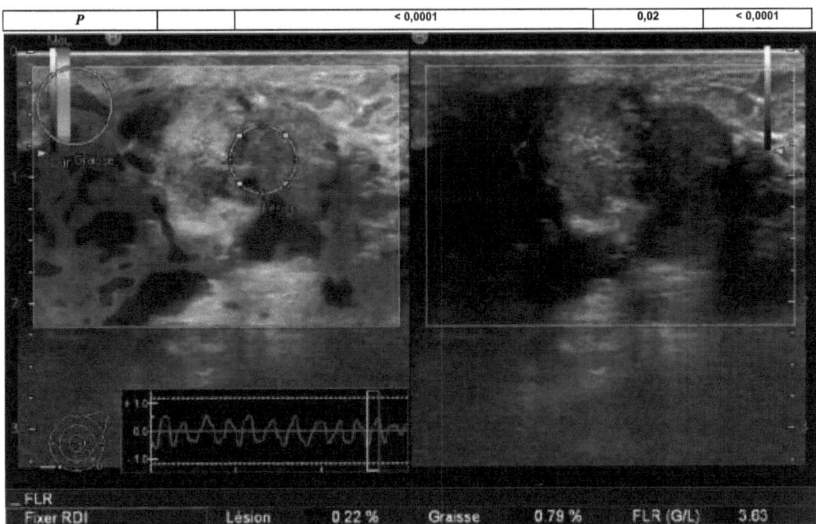

Fig. 53: Papilloma in a 45-year-old woman (a) Elastographic image. Mass with an elasticity score of 3 and an elasticity ratio of 3.63. (b) Ultrasound image. Mass classified as BIRADS 4c.

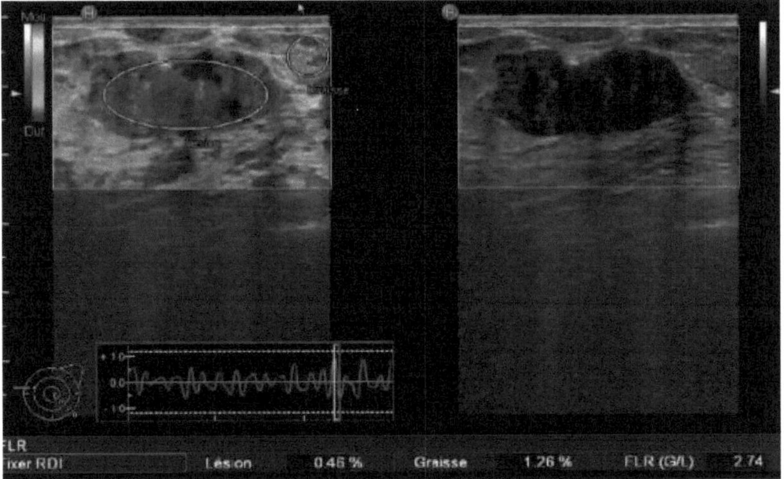

Fig. 54: PASH tumour in a 21-year-old woman. (a) Elastographic image. Mass with an elasticity score of 2 and an elasticity ratio of 2.74. (b) Ultrasound image. Mass classified BI-RADS 4a.

5.6.1.1.1. Fibro-epithelial tumours

The 30 phyllodes tumours studied were classified in colorimetric score 2 in 20 cases (66.7%) and in score 3 in 10 cases (33.3%).

The 189 fibroadenomas studied were classified as colorimetric score 1 in four cases (2.1%), 2 in 139 cases (73.5%), score 3 in 45 cases (23.8%) and one lesion scored

4.

Overall, scores 2 and 3 were most frequently found in both tumour types, with no significant difference *(p = 0.53)*.

The distribution of the elasticity score and the different histological groups according to the amount of stremal cellularity in fibroepithelial tumours are summarised in table 86.

The mean elasticity ratio for the 30 phyllodes was 2.54 + 0.83 and 1.97 + 1.14 for the fibroadenomas. The mean elasticity ratio of the phyllodes was significantly higher than that of the fibroadenomas *(p = 0.001)* (figs. 55 and 56). The elasticity ratios of the different histological groups according to the amount of stremal cellularity are summarised in table 86.

The Spearmans correlation coefficient between the elasticity ratio and the three histological groups according to the amount of stremal cellularity in fibroepithelial tumours was highly significant, with a value of 0.55 *(p < 0.0001)* (figs. 57, 58 and 59).

With regard to the size ratio, there was no significant difference between the two histological types *(p = 0.99)*.

Table 86. Elastography of the different histological groups according to the stremal cellularity of fibroepithelial tumours.

Fibro-epithelial lesions	Not very cellular n = 147	Moderately cellular n = 42	Very cellular n = 30	*P*
Elastography parameters				
Colorimetric score				0,051
1	3 (2,0 %)	1 (2,4 %)	0	
2	116(78,9%)	23 (54,8 %)	20 (66,7 %)	
3	27(18,4%)	18 (42,9,0 %)	10(33,3 %)	
4	1 (0,7 %)	0	0	
Elasticity ratio (mean + standard deviation)	1,88 ± 1,15	2,33 ±1,03	2,53 ±0,83	0,002
Size ratio (mean + standard deviation)	0,99 ±0,031	0,98 ± 0,029	0,97 ± 0,024	0,792

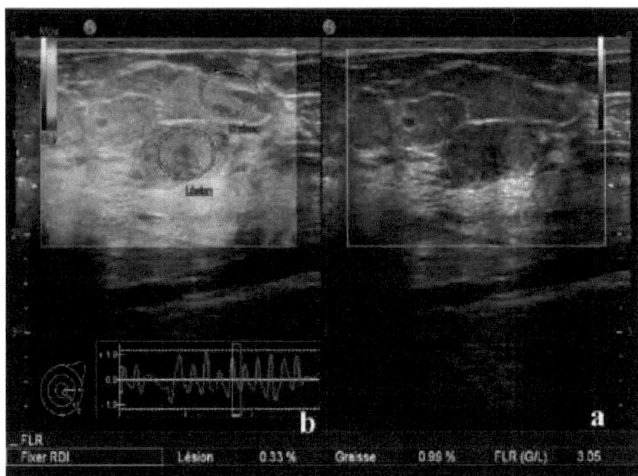

Fig. 55: Phyllodes tumour in a 31-year-old woman. (a) Ultrasound image. Oval-shaped mass with circumscribed contours and a thin interface, classified as BI-RADS 3. (b) Elastographic image. Mass with an elasticity score of 2 and an elasticity ratio of 3.05.

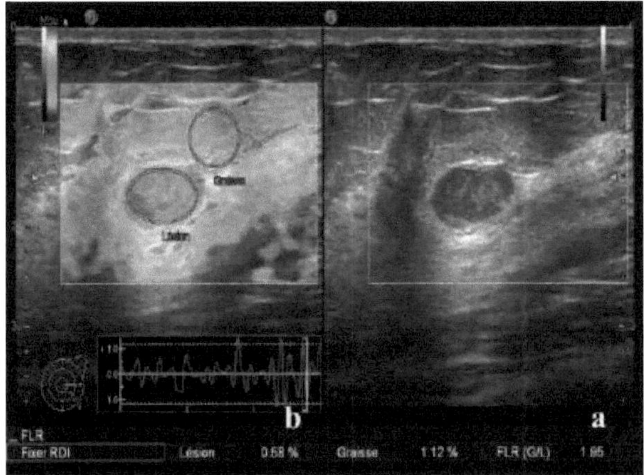

Fig. 56: Fibroadenoma in a 41-year-old woman. (a) Ultrasound image. Oval shaped mass with circumscribed contours and thin interface, classified as BI-RADS 3. (b) Elastographic image. Mass with an elasticity score of 2 and an elasticity ratio of 1.95.

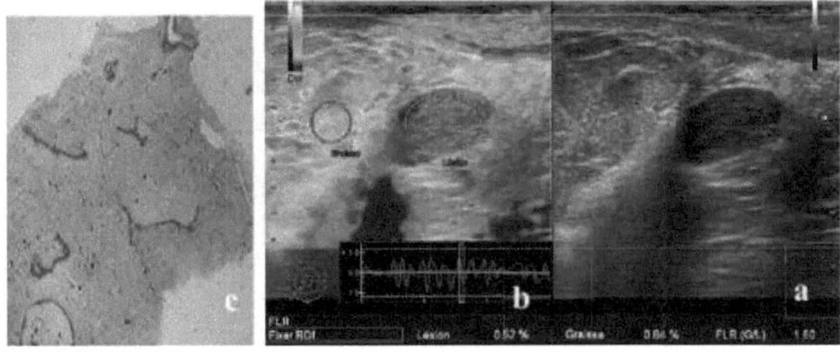

Fig. 57: Fibroadenoma in a 41-year-old woman. (a) Ultrasound image. Oval-shaped mass with circumscribed contours and a thin interface, classified as BI-RADS 3. (b) Elastographic image. Mass with an elasticity score of 2 and an elasticity ratio of 1.60. (c) Histology. Fibroadenoma with myxoid stroma, poorly cellular.

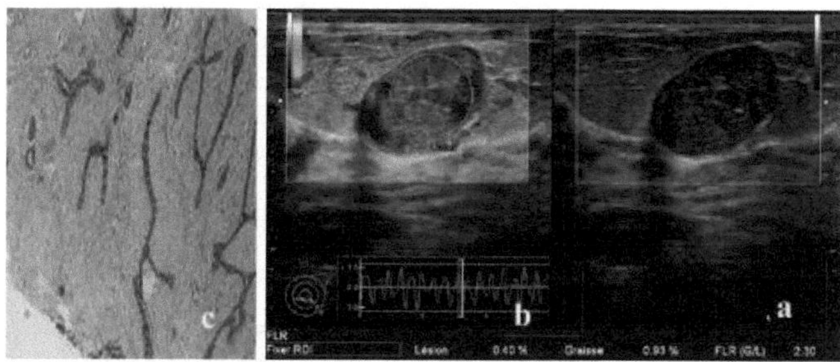

Fig. 58: Fibroadenoma in a 26-year-old woman. (a) Ultrasound image. Oval shaped mass with circumscribed contours and fine interface, classified as BI-RADS 3. (b) Elastographic image. Mass with an elasticity score of 2 and an elasticity ratio of 2.30. (c) Histology. Fibroadenoma with moderately cellular stroma.

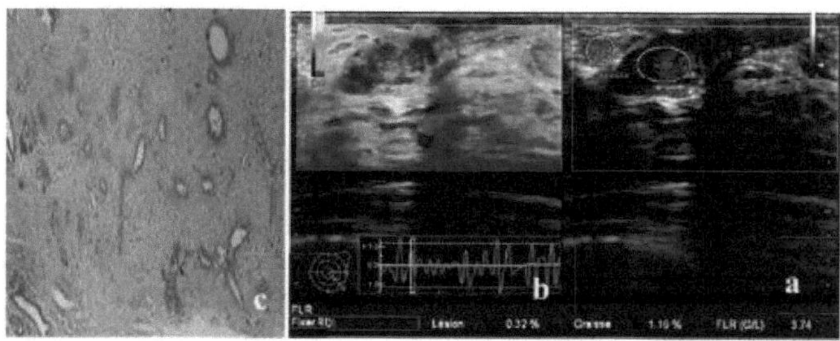

Fig. 59: Phyllodes tumour in a 46-year-old woman. (a) Ultrasound image. Oval-shaped mass with circumscribed contours and thin interface, classified as BI-RADS 3. (b) Elastographic image. Mass with an elasticity score of 3 and an elasticity ratio of 3.74. (c) Histology. Phyllodes tumour with highly cellular stroma.

5.6.1.2. Malignant lesions

Of the 77 malignant lesions, 75 (97.40%) were invasive carcinomas and two were carcinomas in situ (2.60%).

Malignant lesions were more often scored 4 and 5, in 69 cases (89.61%), and eight lesions (2.35%) were scored 2 and 3. These included one lesion of carcinoma in situ, two lesions of infiltrating NST carcinoma, one infiltrating lobular carcinoma and four miscellaneous lesions (intracystic papillary carcinoma, colloid carcinoma, cribriform carcinoma and micro-papillary carcinoma) (tables 87).

The mean elasticity ratio of infiltrating carcinomas was higher than that of carcinomas in situ, respectively 33.30 + 40.24 vs 12.02 + 4.58 ($p < 0.0001$) (figs. 60 and 61).

The mean elasticity ratio for infiltrating lobular carcinomas was higher than for the other histological types, but with no significant difference ($p = 0.16$) (Tables 87) (figs. 62, 63 and 64).

The mean size ratio for invasive lobular carcinomas was significantly higher than for other histological types *(p<0.0001)*.

Table 87. Correlations between histological types of malignant masses and elastographic parameters.

Histological types	**Carcinoma in situ n = 2**	**Invasive carcinoma NST n = 55**	**Invasive lobular carcinoma n = 9**	**Mixed infiltrating carcinoma n = 4**	**Other n = 7**	*P*
Elastography parameters						
Colorimetric score						**< 0,0001**
1	0	0	0	0	0	
2	0	1 (1,8%)	0	0	0	
3	1 (50,0 %)	1 (1,8%)	1 (11,1 %)	0	4 (57,1 %)	
4	1 (50,0 %)	4 (7,3 %)	0	1 (25,0 %)	0	
5	0	49 (98,1 %)	8 (88,9 %)	3 (75,0 %)	3 (42,9 %)	
Elasticity ratio (average + standard deviation)	12,02 + 4,5	34,55 + 40,43	53,40 + 51,81	8,68 + 1,72	11,13 + 10,66	0,16
Size ratio (mean + standard deviation)	1,00 + 0,0	1,21+0,146	1,52 + 0,43	1,22 + 0,11	1,06 + 0,75	**< 0,0001**

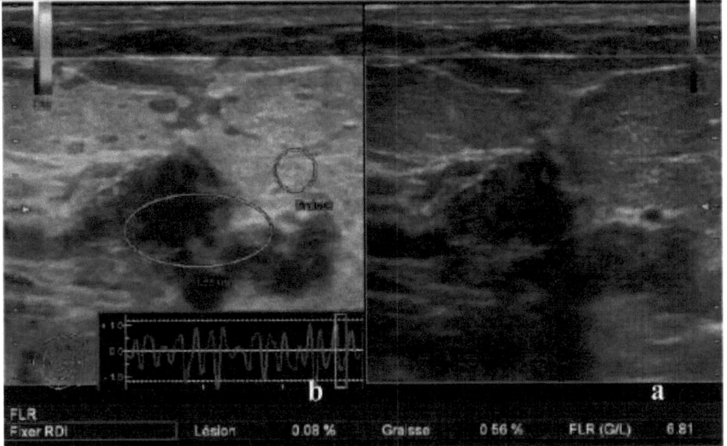

Fig. 60: Carcinoma in situ in a 69-year-old woman (a) Ultrasound image. A mass of irregular shape and contours, with a fine interface, classified as BI-RADS 4c. (b) Elastographic image. Mass with an elasticity score of 5 and an elasticity ratio of 6.81.

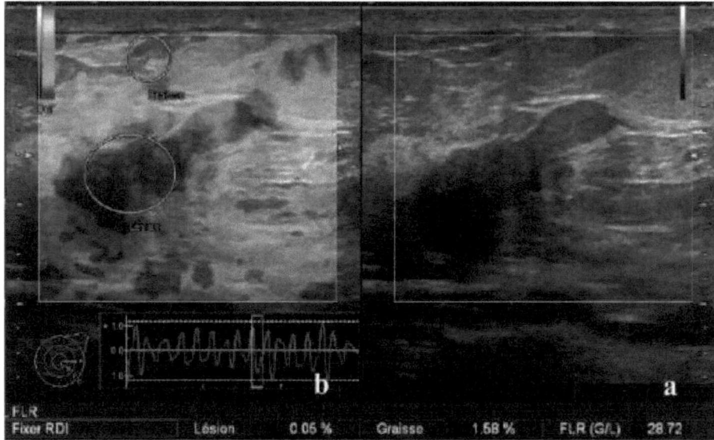

Fig. 61: Infiltrating carcinoma in a 47-year-old woman. Ultrasound image. A mass of irregular shape and contours, with an abrupt interface, classified as BI-RADS 4c. (b) Elastographic image. Mass with an elasticity score of 5 and an elasticity ratio of 28.72.

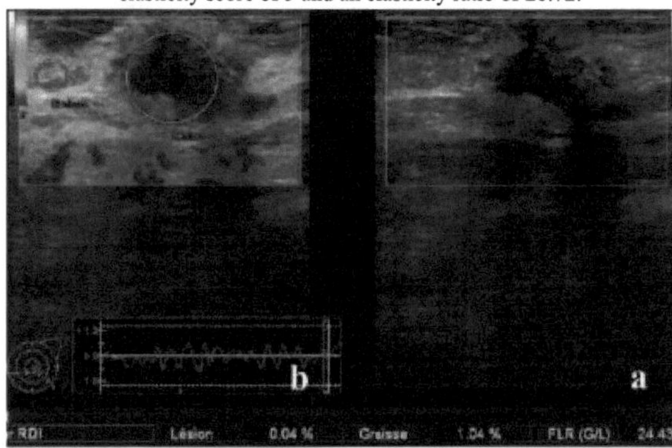

Fig. 62 : NST infllrant carcinoma in a 52-year-old woman. Ultrasound image. Irregularly shaped mass with spiculated contours surrounded by a peripheral echogenic halo, classified as BI-RADS 5. (b) Elastographic image. Mass with an elasticity score of 5, an elasticity ratio of 24.43 and a calculated size ratio of 1.5.

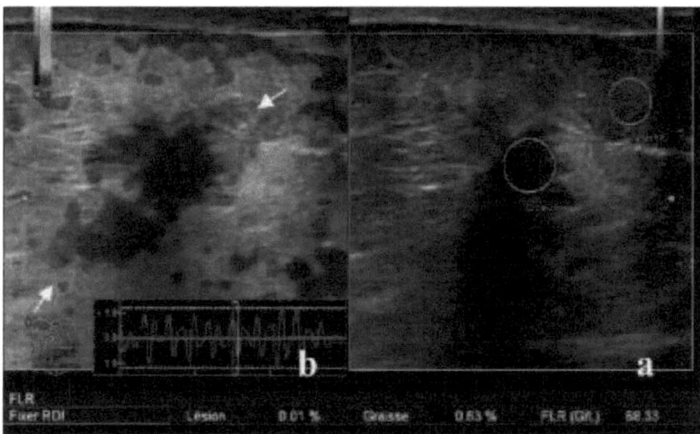

Fig. 63 : Lobular carcinoma in a 48-year-old woman. Ultrasound image. Irregularly shaped mass with spiculated contours and a thin interface, classified as BI-RADS 5. (b) Elastographic image. Mass with an elasticity score of 5, an elasticity ratio of 68.33 and a calculated size ratio of 2.27 (arrows).

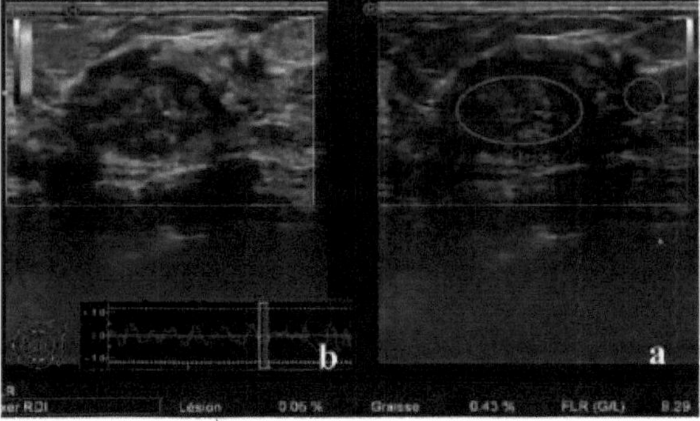

Fig. 64 : Colloid infllrant carcinoma in a 45-year-old woman. Ultrasound image. Oval shaped mass with microlobulated contours and fine interface, classified BI-RADS 4a. (b) Elastographic image. Mass with an elasticity score of 4, an elasticity ratio of 8.29 and a calculated size ratio of 1.

5.6.2. Histopronostic grade

Score 5 was found most often in the different SBR grades, with no significant difference *(p = 0.6)*.

Grade III tumours were significantly associated with highest elasticity ratio values *(p = 0.017)*. The difference in elasticity ratio was greater between grades I and II than between grades II and III (table 88) (figs. 65, 66 and 67).

There was no significant difference in the size ratio between the different histological grades *(p = 0.31)*.

Table 88. Correlations between histological grade and elastographic parameters.

Histopronostic grade	**Grade I n = 7**	**Grade II n = 57**	**Grade III n = ll**	*P*
Elastography parameters				
Colorimetric score				0,26
1	0	0	0	
2	0	0	1 (9,1 %)	
3	1 (14,3 %)	4 (7,0 %)	1 (9,1 %)	
4	1 (14,3%)	4 (7,0 %)	0	
5	5 (71,4%)	49 (86,0 %)	9(81,8 %)	
Elasticity ratio (mean + standard deviation)	10,12 ±5,44	33,10 ±36,55	55,03 ±62,18	**0,017**
Size ratio (mean + standard deviation)	1,15 ± 0,12	1,26 ±0,24	1,17 ± 0,15	0,308

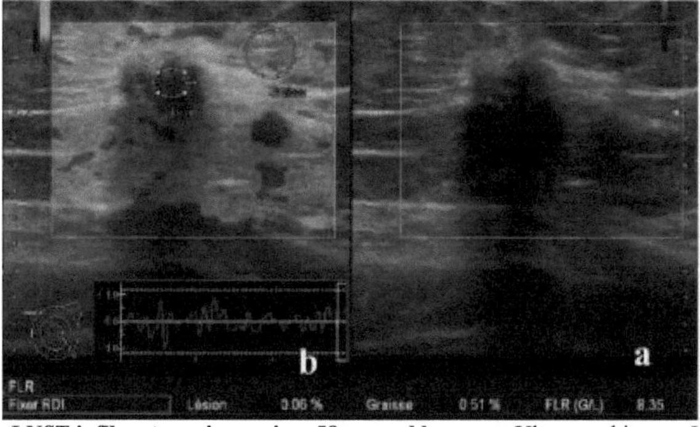

Fig. 65 : Grade I NST infllrant carcinoma in a 58-year-old woman. Ultrasound image. Irregularly shaped mass with spiculated contours, surrounded a peripheral echogenic halo, graded BIRADS 5. (b) Elastographic image. Mass with an elasticity score of 5 and an elasticity ratio of 8.35.

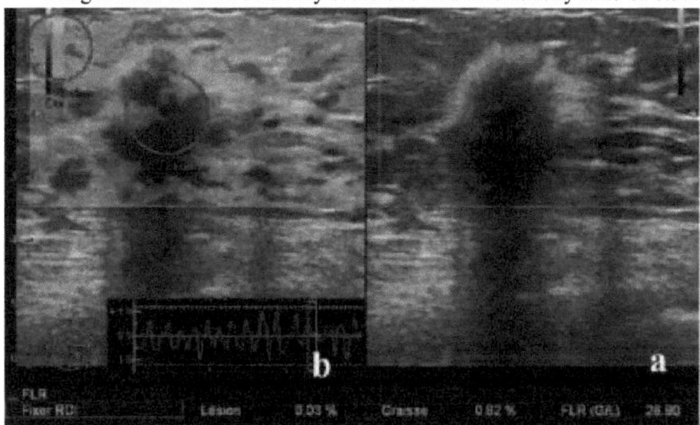

Fig. 66 : Grade II NST infllrant carcinoma in a 45-year-old woman. Ultrasound image. Irregularly shaped mass with spiculated contours, surrounded by a peripheral echogenic halo, graded BIRADS 5. (b) Elastographic image. Mass with an elasticity score of 5 and an elasticity ratio of 26.80.

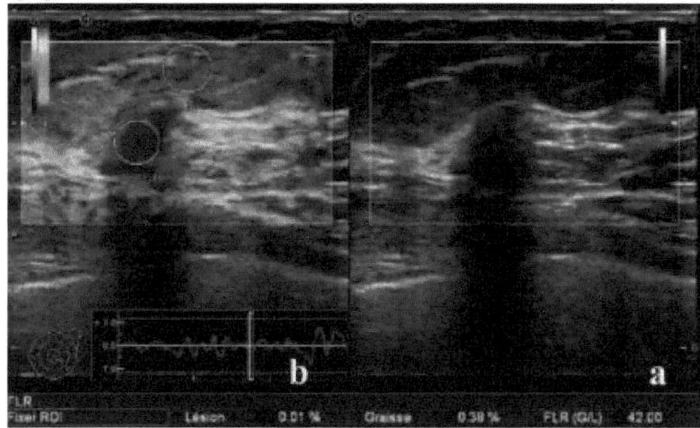

Fig. 67: Grade III NST infllrant carcinoma in a 56-year-old woman. Ultrasound image. Irregularly shaped mass with spiculated contours, surrounded by a peripheral echogenic halo, graded BIRADS 5. (b) Elastographic image. Mass with an elasticity score of 5 and an elasticity ratio of 42.

5.6.3. Hormone receptors

5.6.3.1. Restrogen receptors

Score 5 was found most often, irrespective of the presence or absence of restrogen receptors, with no significant difference *(p = 0.71)*. However, seven lesions scored 2 and 3 were found in the receptor-positive group.

The mean elasticity ratio of receptor-negative lesions was higher than that of receptor-positive lesions, respectively 68.78 + 65.06 vs. 27.15 + 31.23 *(p = 0.001)* (table 89) (figs. 68 and 69).

However, there was no significant difference between the two groups in terms of height ratio *(p = 0.911)*.

Table 89. Correlations between the presence or absence of restrogenic receptors and elastographic parameters.

Mass	Restrogen receptor positive n = 64	Restrogen receptor negative n = ll	P
Elastography parameters			
Colorimetric score			0,71
1	0	0	
2	1 (1,6%)	0	
3	6 (9,4 %)	0	
4	4 (6,3 %)	1 (9,1 %)	
5	53 (82,8 %)	10 (90,9 %)	
Elasticity ratio (mean + standard deviation)	27,15 ±31,23	68,78 ±65,06	**0,001**
Size ratio (mean + standard deviation)	1,24 ±0,23	1,23 ±0,16	0,911

5.6.3.2. Progesterone receptors

In table 90, score 5 was found most often, irrespective of the presence or absence of progesterone receptors, with no significant difference *(p = 0.55)*. However, seven lesions scored 2 and 3 were found in the receptor-positive group.

The mean elasticity ratio of receptor-negative lesions was higher than that of receptor-positive lesions, 57.00 + 60.07 vs 26.81 + 30.64 respectively (p = *0.007*) (figs. 68 and 69).

For the height ratio, there was no significant difference between the two groups *(p = 0.52)*.

Table 90. Correlations between the presence or absence of progesterone receptors and elastographic parameters.

Mass	Progesterone receptor positive n = 59	Negative progesterone receptors n = 16	P
Elastography parameters			
Colorimetric score			0,55
1	**0**	**0**	
2	1(1,7%)	**0**	
3	6 (10,2 %)	**0**	
4	4 (6,8 %)	1 (6,3 %)	

5	48 (81,4%)	15 (93,8 %)	
Elasticity ratio (mean + standard deviation)	26,81 ±30,64	57,00 ± 60,07	**0,007**
Size ratio (mean + standard deviation)	1,24 ±0,24	1,20 ±0,14	0,52

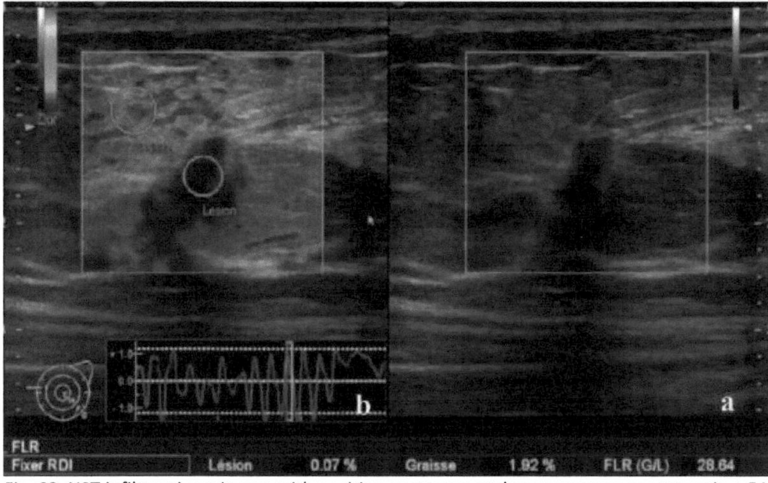

Fig. 68: NST infiltranti carcinoma with positive oestrogen and progesterone receptors in a 54-year-old woman. Ultrasound image. Irregularly shaped mass with spiculated contours, surrounded by a peripheral echogenic halo, classified as BI-RADS 5. (b) Elastographic image. Mass with an elasticity score of 5 and an elasticity ratio of 28.64.

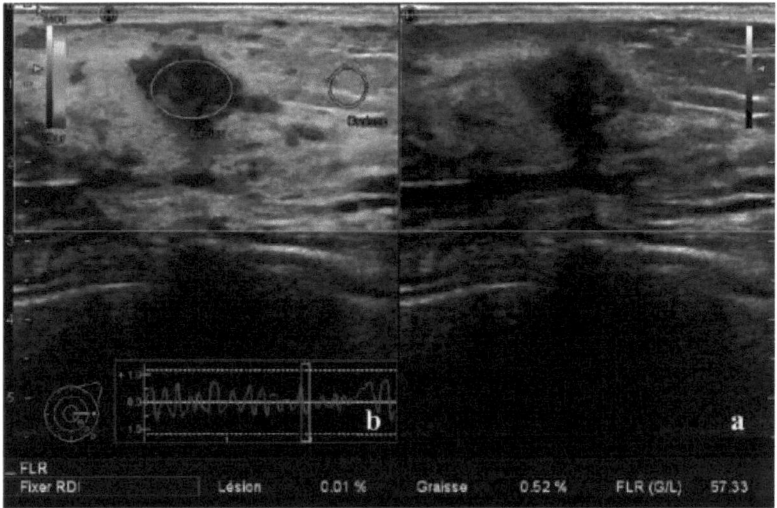

Fig. 69: Invasive NST carcinoma, oestrogen and progesterone receptor negative in a 48-year-old woman. Ultrasound image. Irregularly shaped mass with spiculated contours, surrounded by a peripheral echogenic halo, classified as BI-RADS 5. (b) Elastographic image. Mass with an elasticity score of 5 and an elasticity ratio of 57.33.

As shown in Table 91, score 5 was found in all lesions with HER2 overexpression.

For HER2-negative lesions, scores 4 and 5 were more frequently found. In contrast, seven lesions scored 2 and 3 were found in the HER2-negative group.
The mean elasticity ratio of HER2-positive lesions was higher than that of HER2-negative lesions 54.63 + 30.70 vs 30.70 + 40.71, but with no significant difference *(p = 0.11)*.
For the height ratio, there was no significant difference between the two groups *(p = 0.19)*.

Table 91. Correlations between the presence or absence of HER2 overexpression and elastographic parameters.

Mass	HER2 receptor positive n = 8	HER2 receptor negative n = 67	P
Elastography parameters			
Colorimetric score			0,64
1	0	0	
2	0	1 (1,5 %)	
3	0	6 (9,0 %)	
4	0	5 (7,5 %)	
5	8 (100 %)	55 (82,1 %)	
Elasticity ratio (mean + standard deviation)	54,63 ±30,70	30,70 ±40,71	0,11
Size ratio (mean + standard deviation)	1,14 ±0,08	1,25 ±0,23	0,19

Analysis of table 92 shows no significant difference between the proliferation index (Ki 67) and the elastographic parameters.

Table 92. Correlations between Ki 67 and elastographic parameters.

Mass	Ki 67 <14 n = 14	Ki 67 >14 n = 61	P
Elastography parameters			
Colorimetric score			0,61
1	**0**	**0**	
2	**0**	1 (1,6%)	
3	1 (7,1 %)	5 (8,2 %)	
4	2 (14,3 %)	3 (4,9 %)	
5	11 (78,6%)	52 (85,2 %)	
Elasticity ratio (mean + standard deviation)	27,25 ±38,59	34,63 ±40,84	0,54
Size ratio (mean + standard deviation)	1,24 ±0,26	1,24 ±0,22	0,87

5.6.6. Molecular classification

Among the 75 infiltrating carcinomas, there were 12 masses classified as luminal A (16%), 48 luminal B (64%), 4 luminal B + HER2 (5.33%), 4 HER2 (5.33%) and 7 triple-negative masses (9.33%).
The correlation between elastographic parameters and molecular classification is

shown in Table 93.
The mean elasticity ratio of triple-negative lesions was the highest compared with the other molecular classes. In contrast, the luminal A group had the lowest elasticity ratio values *(p = 0.014)*. Cancers with a high progression potential had a higher lesion hardness (fig. 70).
Score 5 was found most often in the different molecular classes, with no significant difference *(p = 0.69)*. However, seven lesions scored 2 and 3 were found in the B luminal group.
With regard to ce size ratio, there was no significant difference between the different molecular subgroups *(p = 0.52)*.

Table 93. Correlations between molecular classification and elastographic parameters.

Molecular classification	Elastography parameter						
	Elasticity score					Elasticity ratio (average + standard deviation)	Size ratio (average + standard deviation)
	1	2	3	4	5		
Luminal A (n = 12)	0	0	0	2 (16,7%)	10 (83,3%)	18,57 + 11,62	1,27 + 0,27
Luminal B (n = 48)	0	1 (2,1 %)	6 (12,5 %)	2 (4,2%)	39(81,3%)	27,48 + 33,35	1,24 + 0,23
Luminal B + HER2 (n = 4)	0	0	0	0	4 (100%)	48,86 + 40,42	1,13+0,23
HER2 (n = 4)	0	0	0	0	4 (100 %)	60,41+21,81	1,15+ 0,11
Triple negative (n = 7)	0	0	0	1 (14,3%)	6 (85,7%)	73,56 + 82,11	1,27 + 0,17
P	0,69					**0,014**	0,731

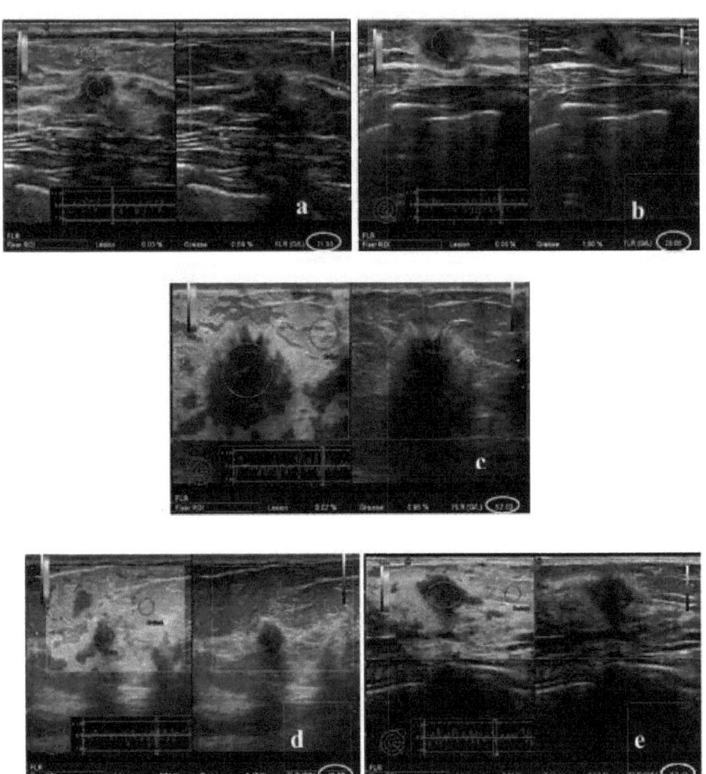

Fig. 70: Invasive carcinoma-like lesions NST. (a) luminal A. (b) Luminal B. (c) Luminal B + HER2. (d) HER2. (e) Triple negative. Elastographic image. All lesions have an elasticity score of 5, but different elasticity ratios. Tumours with high progressive potential (HER2 and Triple negative) had higher elasticity ratio values than tumours with low progressive potential (Luminal A and Luminal B).

5.6.7 Vascular emboli

In the 36 malignant masses operated on, the mean elasticity ratio of lesions with vascular emboli was higher than that of masses without vascular emboli *(p = 0.048)* (fig. 71).

Score 5 was found most often in both groups, with no significant difference *(p = 0.72).* On the other hand, three lesions with a score of 3 were found in the group that no vascular emboli in the operative parts.

mean height ratio showed no significant difference between the two groups *(p = 0.81).*

The correlation between elastographic parameters and the presence of vascular emboli is shown in Table 94.

Table 94. Correlations between the presence of vascular emboli and elastographic parameters.

Mass	**Vascular emboli n = 3**	**No vascular emboli n = 33**	*P*
Elastography parameters			
Colorimetric score			0,72
1	0	0	
2	0	0	
3	0	3 (9,1 %)	
4	0	3 (9,1 %)	
5	3 (100 %)	27 (81,8%)	
Elasticity ratio (mean + standard deviation)	72,62 ± 72,49	29,85 ±30,70	**0,048**
Size ratio (mean + standard deviation)	1,18 ±0,47	1,22 ±0,23	0,807

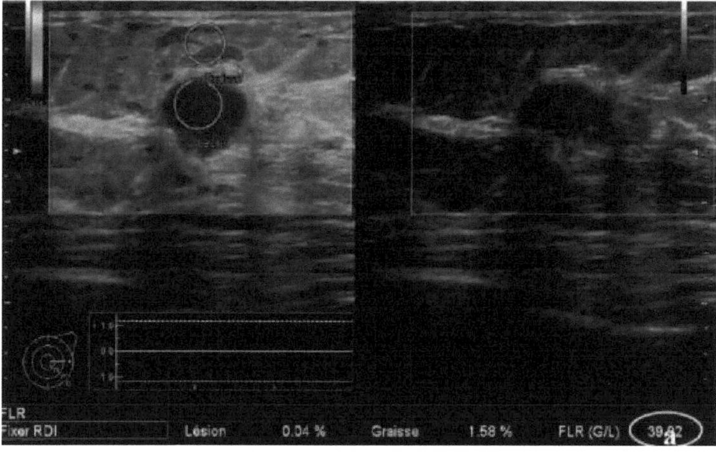

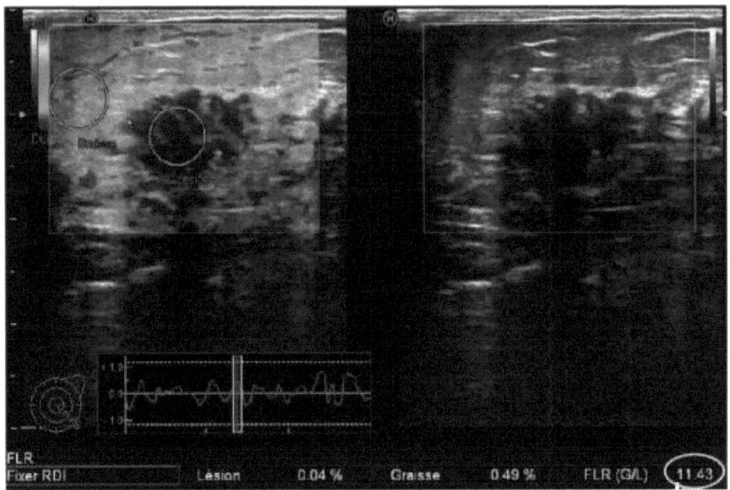

Fig. 71: Vascular emboli. (a) Presence of vascular emboli in the surgical specimen. (b) Absence of vascular emboli in the surgical specimen. Two lesions of NST infiltrating carcinoma type, grade II and luminal type B. The mass with vascular emboli had a higher elasticity ratio value than the mass without vascular emboli.

Analysis of Table 95 showed no significant difference between the presence or absence of necrosis and the elastographic parameters (for all parameters p > 0.05).

Table 95. Correlations between the presence or absence of necrosis and elastographic parameters.

Mass	Necrosis n = 3	No necrosis n = 32	P
Elastography parameters			
Colorimetric score			0,38
1	0	0	
2	0	0	
3	1 (25,0 %)	2 (6,3 %)	
4	0	3 (9,4 %)	
5	3 (75,0 %)	27 (84,4 %)	
Elasticity ratio (mean + standard deviation)	45,27 ±35,13	31,93 ±36,53	0,49
Size ratio (mean + standard deviation)	1,07 ±0,06	1,23 ±0,23	0,188

5.6.9. Fibrosis

The mean elasticity ratio increased in proportion to the abundance of malignant tumour reaction stroma (*p = 0.002*). The Spearmans correlation coefficient between the elasticity ratio and the three groups according to the abundance of fibro-hyaline tumour stroma was highly significant, with a value of 0.50 *(p = 0.005)*. The elasticity ratios of the different groups according to the abundance of fibro-hyaline tumour stroma are summarised in Table 96.

Score 5 was found most frequently in the different groups according to the abundance of reaction stroma, without significant difference *(p = 0.52)*. However, three lesions with a score of 3 were found in the less abundant tumour stroma group (table 96).

The mean height ratio showed no significant difference between the different groups *(p = 0.94)*.

Table 96. Correlations between fibrosis abundance and elastographic parameters.

Fibrosis	**Slightly inconsistent n = 12**	**Moderately rounded n = 20**	**Very inconsistent n = 4**	*P*
Elastography parameters				
Colorimetric score				0,07
1	0	0	0	
2	0	0	0	
3	3 (25,0 %)	0	0	
4	0	3 (15,0 %)	0	
5	9 (75,0 %)	17 (85,0 %)	4 (100 %)	
Elasticity ratio (mean + standard deviation)	16,55+ 20,61	33,08 + 30,30	85,71 + 55,48	**0,002**
Size ratio (mean + standard deviation)	1,22 + 0,20	1,22 + 0,27	1,18 + 0,072	0,94

5.6.10. Metastatic lymph nodes

The mean elasticity ratio of lesions with lymph node involvement was higher than that of lesions without metastatic lymph nodes, respectively 39.87 + 40.30 vs 25.60 + 29.61, but with no significant difference *(p = 0.23)*.

The other parameters (elasticity score and size ratio) showed no significant difference between the metastatic and non-metastatic groups (table 97).

Table 97. Correlations between lymph node involvement and elastographic parameters.

Weights	**Metastatic lymph n = 19**	**Non-metastatic lymph n = 18**	*P*
Elastography parameters			
Colorimetric score			0,52
1	0	0	
2	0	0	
3	1 (5,3 %)	2(11,1 %)	
4	3 (15,8 %)	1 (5,6 %)	
5	15 (78,9 %)	15 (83,3 %)	
Elasticity ratio (mean + standard deviation)	39,87 ±40,30	25,60 ±29,61	0,23
Size ratio (mean + standard deviation)	1,22 + 0,28	1,21 ±0,23	0,66

5.6.11. Histological size

We were able to measure the histological size of the 37 malignant lesions on the surgical specimens.

For these lesions, the histological size was closer to the elastographic size (respectively 27.03 + 15.35 mm vs 27.26 + 13.63 mm) than to the ultrasound size (23.21 + 11.97 mm) (table 98).

Table 98. Comparison between histological size, ultrasound size and elastographic size.		
Mass n = 37	**Average size in mm (mean + standard deviation)**	***P***
Histology	27,03 + 15,35	-
Ultrasound	23,21 ±11,97	0,23
Elastography	27,26+ 13,63	0,96

6. Diagnostic performance

6.1. Diagnostic performance of ultrasound

Ultrasound diagnostic performance, considering masses classified as BI-RADS 3 as benign (negative examination) and masses classified as BI-RADS 4 and 5 as malignant (positive examination), showed a sensitivity of 100% (77/77). On the other hand, specificity and positive predictive value (PPV) were poor, respectively 25.5% (76/298) and 25.75% (77/299), for a negative predictive value (NPV) of 100% (76/76) (tables 99 and 100). 74.25% (222/299) of false-positives were found, with 220 benign lesions classified as BI-RADS 4 and two lesions classified as BI-RADS 5. The histology of the two false-positive lesions classified as BI-RADS 5 corresponded to a granulomatous mastitis lesion and a cytosteatonecrosis lesion. There were no false-negatives on ultrasound.

Table 99. Distribution of benign and malignant masses according to the diagnostic performance of ultrasound.		
Mass	**Malignant n = 77**	**Benign n = 298**
Positive ultrasound (BI-RADS > 4a)	**Real positives**	**False positives**
	77	**222**
Ultrasound negative (BI-RADS = 3)	**False negatives**	**True negatives**
	0	**76**

Table 100. Diagnostic performance of ultrasound.						
	AUC	**Sensitivity**	**Specific**	**VPP**	**VPN**	**Accuracy**
Ultrasound mode B						
Categories BI-RADS US > 4a [Confidence interval 95% (CI 95%)].	0,628 [0,566-0,689]	100% [95,25-100]	25,5 % [20,9-30,7%]	25,75 % [21,1-31%]	100 % [95,2-100]	40,8 % [35,9-45,8%]

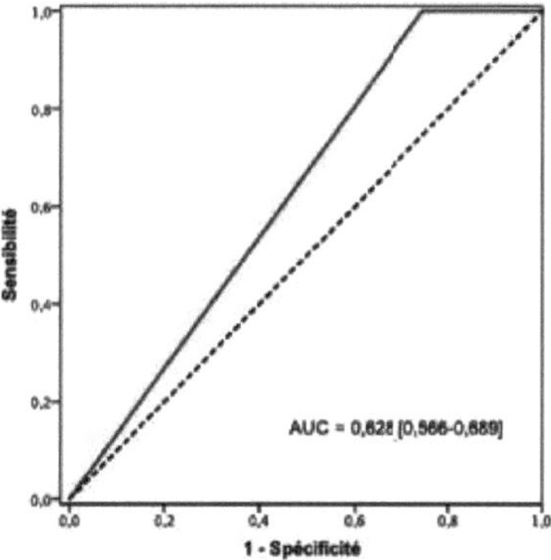

Fig. 72. ROC curve for B-mode ultrasound. AUC of 0.628.

6.2. Diagnostic performance of elastography

The diagnostic performance of the elasticity score (masses scored 1, 2 and 3 were considered benign [negative examination] and masses scored 4 and 5 malignant [positive examination], table 101) showed a sensitivity of 89,61% (69/77), a specificity of 97.65% (291/298), a positive predictive value (PPV) of 90.79% (69/76), a negative predictive value (NPV) of 97.32% (291/299) and an accuracy of 96% (360/375) (table 104).

The diagnostic performance of the elasticity ratio for a best estimated threshold value of 3.67, shows a sensitivity of 96.1% (74/77), a specificity of 93.29% (278/298), a positive predictive value (PPV) of 78.72% (74/94), a negative predictive value (NPV) of 98.93% (278/281) and an accuracy of 93.87% (352/375) (tables 102 and 104).

With a best calculated cut-off value of 1.045, the size ratio shows a sensitivity of 87.01% (67/77), a specificity of 93.29% (292/298), a positive predictive value (PPV) of 91.78% (67/73), a negative predictive value (NPV) of 96.69% (292/302) and an accuracy of 95.73% (359/375) (tables 103 and 104).

Table 101. Distribution of benign and malignant masses according to the diagnostic performance of the elasticity score.

Mass	**Malignant η = 77**	**Benign η = 298**
Positive elasticity score (Score > 4)	**Real positives**	**False positives**
	69	**7**
Negative elasticity score (Score < 4)	**False negatives**	**True negatives**
	8	**291**

Table 102. Distribution benign and malignant masses according to the diagnostic performance of the elasticity ratio.

Mass	**Malignant η = 77**	**Benign n = 298**
Positive elasticity ratio (Ratio>	**Real positives**	**False positives**

3.67)	74	20
Negative elasticity ratio (Ratio < 3.67)	False negatives	True negatives
	3	278

Table 103. Distribution of benign and malignant masses according to the diagnostic performance of the size ratio.

Mass	Malignant n = 77	Benign n = 298
Positive size ratio (Ratio > 1.045)	Real positives	False positives
	67	6
Negative size ratio (Ratio < 1.045)	False negatives	True negatives
	10	292

Table 104. Diagnostic performance of elastographic parameters.

	AUC	Sensitivity	Specific	VPP	VPN	Accuracy
Elastography						
Elasticity score >4 [95% CI]	0,936 [0,895-0,977]	89,61% [82,8-94,6]	97,65% [95,2-98,9]	90,79% [82,2-95,5]	97,32% [94,8-98,6]	96% [93.5-98,6]
Elasticity ratio >3.67 [CI 95%].	0,947 [0,917-0,977]	96,1% [89,2-98,7]	93,29% [89,9-95,6]	78,72% [69,4-85,8]	98,93% [96,9-99,6]	93,87% [90,9-95,9]
P	**0,67**	0,21	**0,003**	**0,04**	0,26	0,9
Size ratio > 1.045 [95% CI].	0,925 [0,880-0,970]	87,01% [77,7-92,8]	97,99% [95,7-99,1]	91,78% [83,2-96,2]	96,69% [94,1-98,2]	95,73% [93,2-97,4]
P	0,72	0,08	**0,008**	**0,03**	0,12	0,76

The *dep* values indicate comparisons between the elasticity score/elasticity ratio and the elasticity ratio/size ratio.

The performance of the elasticity score and size ratio were significantly better in terms of specificity and PPV than the elasticity ratio *(p < 0.05)*. However, the elasticity ratio showed better sensitivity and NPV compared with the other two parameters, but with no significant difference *(p > 0.05)*. In terms of ROC curves, the elasticity ratio had the largest area under the curve (AUC) compared with the other two elastographic parameters, but with no significant difference *(p = 0.74)* (fig. 73).
A strong correlation was found between the score and the elasticity ratio (Spearman correlation coefficient = 0.77,^ < *0.0001*). Similarly, a strong correlation was found between the elasticity score and the height ratio, but also between the elasticity and height ratios (Spearman correlation coefficient = 0.53,j9 < *0.0001* and Pearson correlation coefficient = 0.50,^ < *0.0001* respectively*)*.

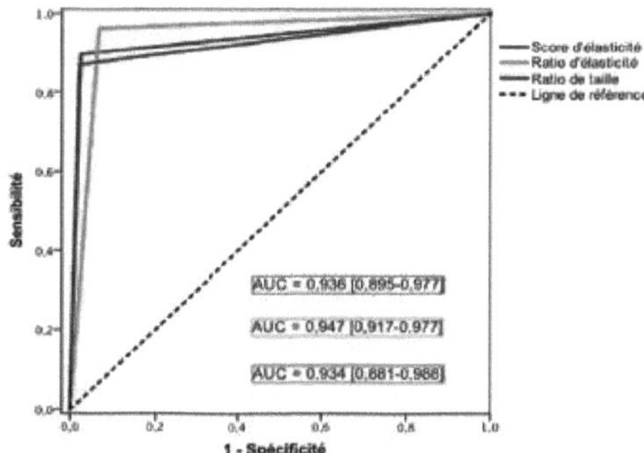

Fig. 73. ROC curve of elastographic parameters

6.2.1. False negatives

In the elastographic colorimetric score, there y were eight false-negatives, i.e. 2.68% of negative results. The histology corresponded to three infiltrating NST carcinomas, one cribriform carcinoma, one micro-papillary carcinoma, one intracystic papillary carcinoma, one colloid carcinoma and one ductal carcinoma in situ. These false negatives were initially classified on ultrasound in two cases as BI-RADS 4a, in two other cases as BI-RADS 4b and in four cases as BI-RADS 4c (figs. 74 and 75).

Using a cut-off value of 3.67 for the elasticity ratio, there were three false negatives (1.07%). The histology of the three false negatives was an infiltrating NST carcinoma, a micro-papillary carcinoma and an intracystic papillary carcinoma. These false-negatives had initially been classified by ultrasound in the three BI-RADS 4 cases (fig. 75).

With regard to the size ratio, for a cut-off value of 1.045, there were ten false negatives (3.31%). The histology corresponded to five infiltrating NST carcinomas, one cribriform carcinoma, one papillary intracystic carcinoma, one colloid carcinoma and two intracanal carcinomas. These false negatives had initially been classified on ultrasound in one case as BI-RADS 4a, in four cases as BI-RADS 4b, in four other cases as BI-RADS 4c and in one case as BI-RADS 5 (fig. 74).

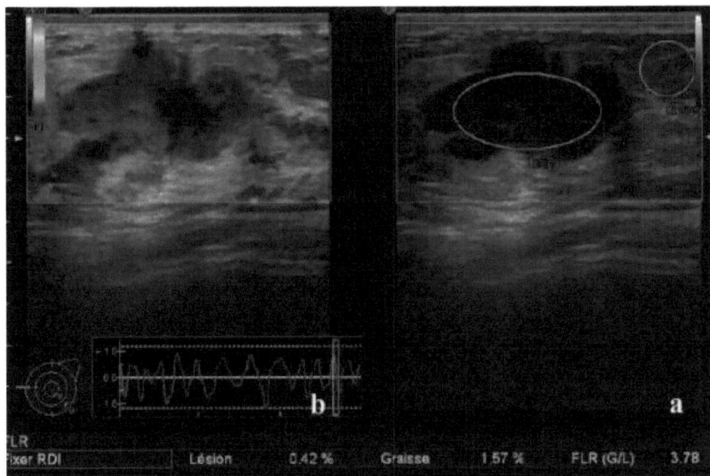

Fig. 74: **Grade III infiltranous lobular carcinoma in a 43-year-old woman.** (a) Ultrasound image. Oval-shaped mass with microlobulated contours and abrupt interface, classified BI-RADS 4a. (b) Elastographic image. Mass with an elasticity score of 2, a calculated elasticity ratio of 3.78 and a size ratio of 1.

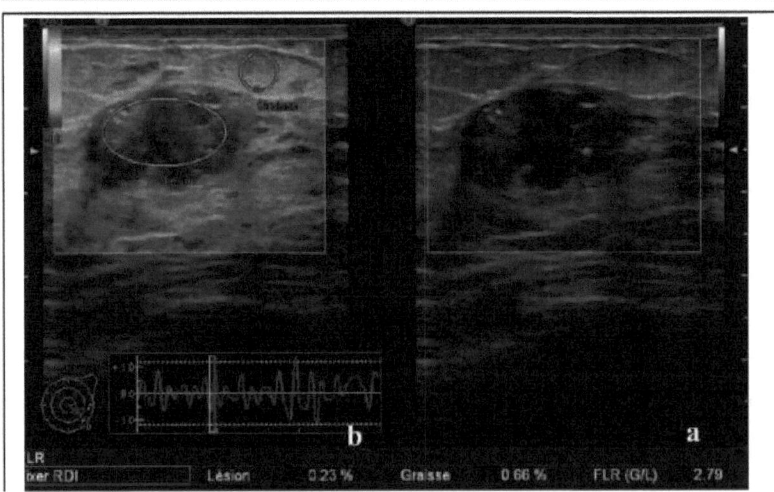

Fig. 75: **Grade II infiltrating micropapillary carcinoma in a 46-year-old woman.** (a) Ultrasound image. Oval-shaped mass with irregular contours and abrupt interface, classified BI-RADS 4c. (b) Elastographic image. Mass with an elasticity score of 3, a calculated elasticity ratio of 2.79 and a claculated size ratio of 1.1.

6.2.2. False positives

When the elasticity score was taken into account, there were seven false positives, representing 6.8% of positive results. The histology corresponded to two granulomatous mastitis (one BI-RADS 4c, one BI-RADS 5), two cytosteatonecroses (one BI-RADS 4a and one BI-RADS 4c), two adenomyo-epitheliomas (two BI-RADS 4a), one fibroadenoma fibrous (BI-RADS 4a) (figs. 76

and 77).

For the elasticity ratio, there were 20 false negatives (21.28%). The histology of the 20 false positives was nine fibroadenomas (three BI-RADS 3, six BI-RADS 4a), three phyllodes tumours (one BI-RADS 3, two BI-RADS 4a), three fibrocystic mastopathies (three BI-RADS 4a), one adenomyo-epithelioma (BIRADS 4a), two granulomatous mastitises (one BI-RADS 4c, one BI-RADS 5), one cytosteatonecrosis lesion (BI-RADS 4c) and one epidermal cyst (BIRADS 3) (figs. 76 and 77).

Six benign lesions were false positive (8.22%) taking into account the size ratio. The histology of the six false positives corresponded to three granulomatous mastitis lesions (two BI-RADS 4c and one BI-RADS 5), one adenomyo-epithelioma (BI-RADS 4a), one cytostéatonécrose (BI-RADS 4c) and one abscess (BIRADS 4c) (figs. 76 and 78).

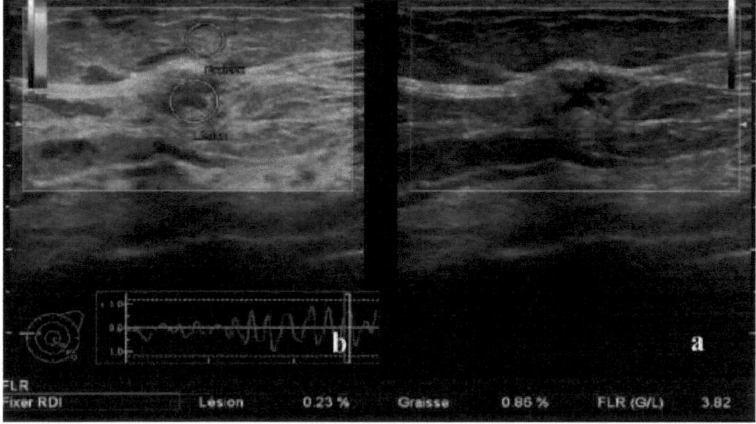

Fig. 76: Granulomatous mastitis in a 48-year-old woman. (a) Ultrasound image. Irregularly shaped mass with spiculated contours, surrounded by a peripheral echogenic halo, classified as BI-RADS 5. (b) Elastographic image. Mass with an elasticity score of 5 and an elasticity ratio of 3.82, above the threshold value, and a calculated size ratio of 1.2.

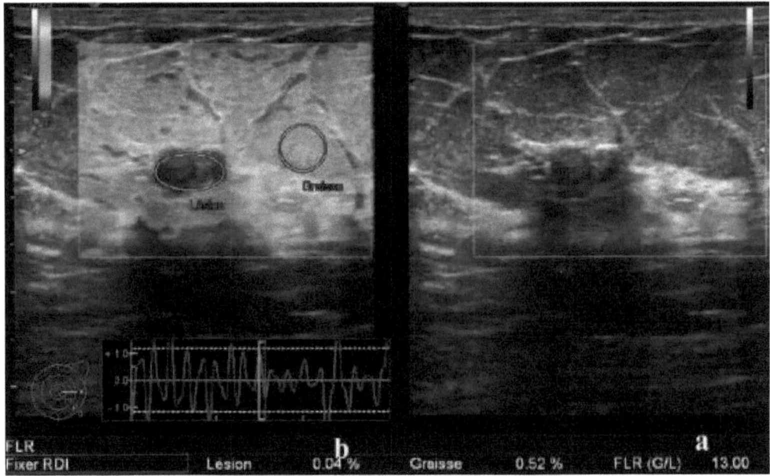

Fig. 77: Fibroadenoma fibreux in a 61-year-old woman. (a) Ultrasound image. Oval shaped mass with microlobulated contours, abrupt interface, isoechoic, classified BI-RADS 4a. (b) Elastographic image. Mass with an elasticity score of 4, an elasticity ratio of 13 and a size ratio of 1.

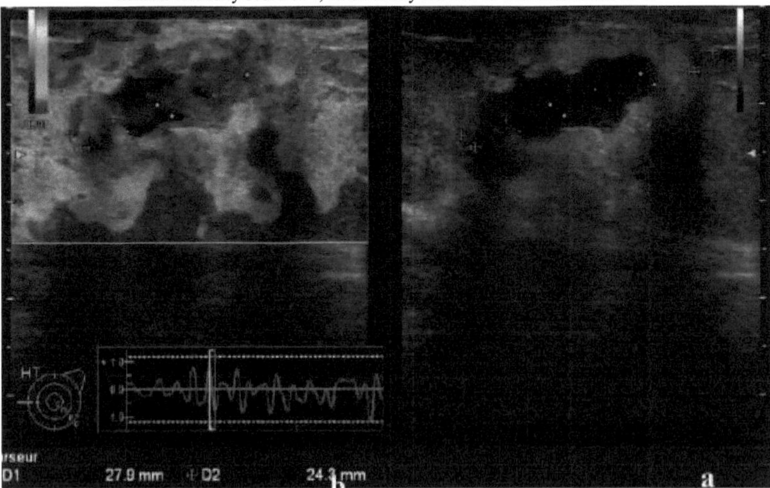

Fig. 78: Granulomatous mastitis in a 43-year-old woman. (a) Ultrasound image. Mass of irregular shape and contours, surrounded by a peripheral echogenic halo, classified BI-RADS 4c. (b) Elastographic image. Mass with an elasticity score of 2 and a calculated size ratio of 1.12.

6.3. Diagnostic performance of elastographic parameters and B-mode ultrasound.

As a reminder, the performances of the different elastographic parameters were compared with B-mode ultrasound. The performance values of B mode ultrasound and the three elastographic parameters in the diagnosis of benign and malignant breast masses are reported in Table 105.

Table 105. Diagnostic performance of ultrasound and elastographic parameters.

	AUC	Sensitivity	Specific	VPP	VPN	Accuracy

Ultrasound mode B						
Categories BI-RADS US > 4a [CI 95%]	0,628 [0,566-0,689]	100 % [95,25-100]	25,5 % [20,9-30,7%]	25,75 % [21,1-31%]	100 % [95,2-100]	40,8 % [35,9-45,8%]
Elastography						
Elasticity score (SE) > 4 [95% CI]	0,936 [0,895-0,977]	89,61% [82,8-94,6]	97,65% [95,2-98,9]	90,79% [82,2-95,5]	97,32% [94,8-98,6]	96% [93.5-98,6]
P	< 0,0001	0,01	< 0,0001	< 0,0001	0,32	< 0,0001
Elasticity ratio (ER) >3.67 [95% CI].	0,947 [0,917-0,977]	96,1% [89,2-98,7]	93,29% [89,9-95,6]	78,72% [69,4-85,8]	98,93% [96,9-99,6]	93,87% [90,9-95,9]
P	< 0,0001	0,24	< 0,0001	< 0,0001	0,84	< 0,0001
Size ratio (SR) > 1.045 [95% CI].	0,925 [0,880-0,970]	87,01% [77,7-92,8]	97,99% [95,7-99,1]	91,78% [83,2-96,2]	96,69% [94,1-98,2]	95,73% [93,2-97,4]
P	< 0,0001	0,003	< 0,0001	< 0,0001	0,23	< 0,0001

***P* values indicate comparisons between B-mode ultrasound and elastographic parameters, [95% Confidence Interval (95% CI)].**

When B-mode ultrasound diagnostic performance values, elasticity score, elasticity ratio and size ratio were compared, all elastography parameters had significantly higher specificity, negative predictive value (PPV) and accuracy than B-mode ultrasound *(p<0.0001).*

The elasticity ratio had equivalent sensitivity to B-mode ultrasound *(p = 0.24).* However, the elasticity score and size ratio had low sensitivity compared with B-mode ultrasound (respectively,^ = *0.01 andp = 0.003).*

In terms of the area under the curve (AUC), the three elastographic parameters had a significantly wider AUC than that of the B-mode ultrasound *(p< 0.0001).*

6.4. Diagnostic performance of combinations of B-mode ultrasound and various elastographic parameters.

As a reminder, the performances of the different combinations B-mode ultrasound and elastographic parameters were compared with B-mode ultrasound alone. The performance values of the ultrasound-elastography combinations in the characterisation of benign and malignant breast masses are reported in Table 106.

Table 106. Diagnostic performance of combinations of ultrasound and elastographic parameters.

	AUC	Sensitivity	Specific	VPP	VPN	Accuracy
Ultrasound mode B						
US mode B [IC 95%]	0,628 [0,566-0,689]	100 % [95,25-100]	25,5 % [20,9-30,7%]	25,75 % [21,1-31%]	100 % [95,2-100]	40,8 % [35,9-45,8%]
Ultrasound + Elastography						
US mode B + SE [IC 95%]	0,936 [0,895-0,977]	89,61% [82,8-94,6]	97,65% [95,2-98,9]	90,79% [82,2-95,5]	97,32% [94,8-98,6]	96% [93.5-98,6]
P	< 0,0001	0,01	< 0,0001	< 0,0001	0,32	< 0,0001
US mode B + SE + RE [IC 95%]	0.940 [0.899-0.980]	89.61% [80.82-94.64]	98.32% [96.13-99.28]	93.23% [85.14-97.08]	97.34% [94.84-97.08]	96.53% [94.16-97.96]
P	< 0,0001	0,01	< 0,0001	< 0,0001	0,32	< 0,0001
US mode B + SE + RE + RT [IC 95%]	0,909 [0,859-0,959]	83,12% [73,23-89,86]	98,66% [96,6-99,48]	94,12% [85,83-97,69]	95,77% [92,89-97,51]	95,47% [92,86-97,15]
P	< 0,0001	0,0005	< 0,0001	< 0,0001	0,14	< 0,0001

The *p-values* indicate comparisons between ultrasound mode B and the various ultrasound-elastography combinations.

The combined use of the B mode ultrasound elasticity score significantly improved AUC from 0.628 to 0.936 *($p < 0.0001$)*, specificity from 25.5% to 97.65% *($p < 0.0001$)*, WP from 25.75% to 90.79% *($p < 0.0001$)* and accuracy from 40.8% to 96% *($p < 0.0001$)*, but with a loss of sensitivity from 100% to 89.61% *($p = 0.01$)*.
Adding the elasticity ratio to the elasticity score-ultrasound mode B combination increased the AUC from 0.628 to 0.940 *($p < 0.0001$)*, specificity from 25.5% to 98.32% *($p < 0.0001$)*, PPV from 25.75% to 93.23% *($p < 0.0001$)* and accuracy from 40.8% to 96.53% *($p < 0.0001$)*, but with a loss of sensitivity from 100% to 89.61% *($p = 0.01$)*.
The combination of B mode ultrasound and the three elastographic parameters very significantly improved specificity over the other combinations from 25.5% to 98.66% *($p < 0.0001$)* and WP from 25.75% to 94.12% *($p < 0.0001$)*. However, there was a significant loss of sensitivity from 100% to 83.12% *($p = 0.0005$)*.

6.4.1. False positives and false negatives

Considering the best performing combination which combines the three elastographic parameters with B mode ultrasound, there are only four false positives andl3 false negatives.
Four false-positives, i.e. 5.88% of positive results. The histology corresponded to two granulomatous mastitis (one BI-RADS 4c, one BI-RADS 5), one cytosteatonecrosis lesion (BI-RADS 4c) and one adenomyo-epithelioma (BI-RADS 4a) (fig.79 and 80).
13 false-negatives (4.23%). Histology corresponded to seven infiltrating NST carcinomas, one cribriform carcinoma, one papillary intracystic carcinoma, one colloid carcinoma, one micropappillary carcinoma and two intracanal carcinomas. These false negatives had initially been classified in B mode ultrasound in two cases BI-RADS 4a, in five cases BI-RADS 4b, in five cases BI-RADS 4c and BI-RADS 5 in one case (fig. 81).

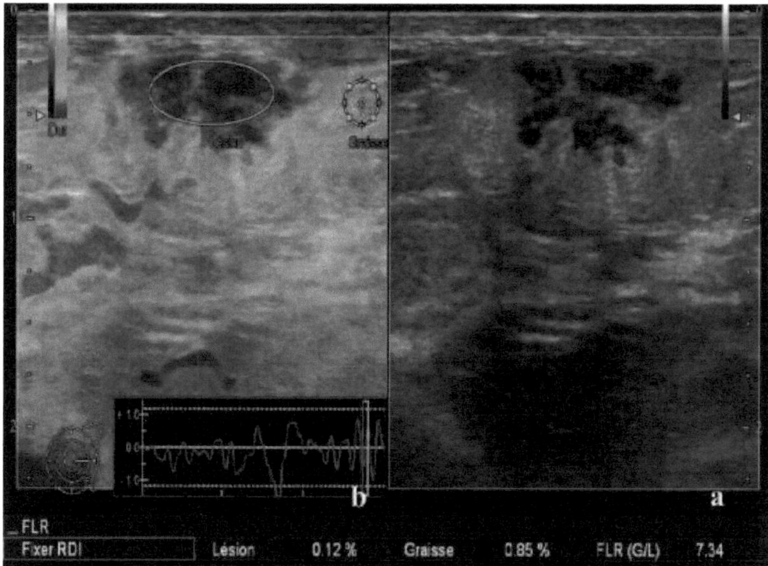

Fig. 79: Granulomatous mastitis in a 53-year-old woman. (a) Ultrasound image. Mass of irregular shape and contours, surrounded a peripheral echogenic halo, classified BI-RADS 4c. (b) Elastographic image. Mass with an elasticity score of 5, an elasticity ratio of 7.34 and a calculated size ratio of 1.45.

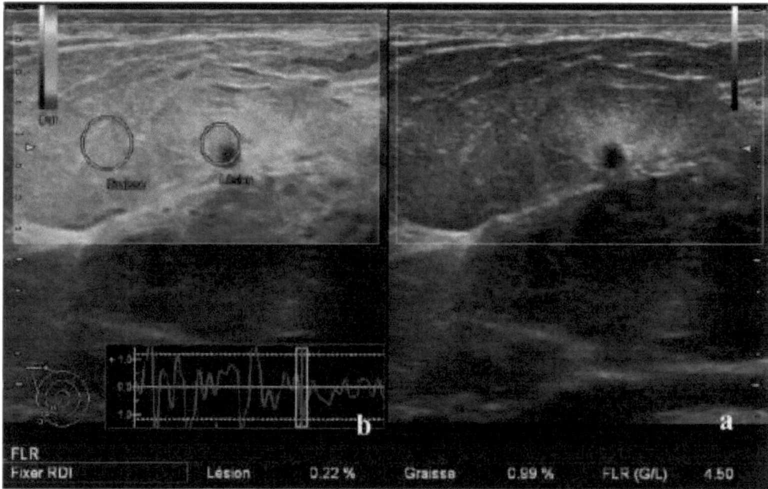

Fig. 80: A cytosteatonecrosis lesion in a 44-year-old woman. (a) Ultrasound image. A round mass with indistinct contours, surrounded by a peripheral echogenic halo, classified as BI-RADS 4c. (b) Elastographic image. Mass with an elasticity score of 4c, an elasticity ratio of 4.5 and a calculated fault ratio of 1.3.

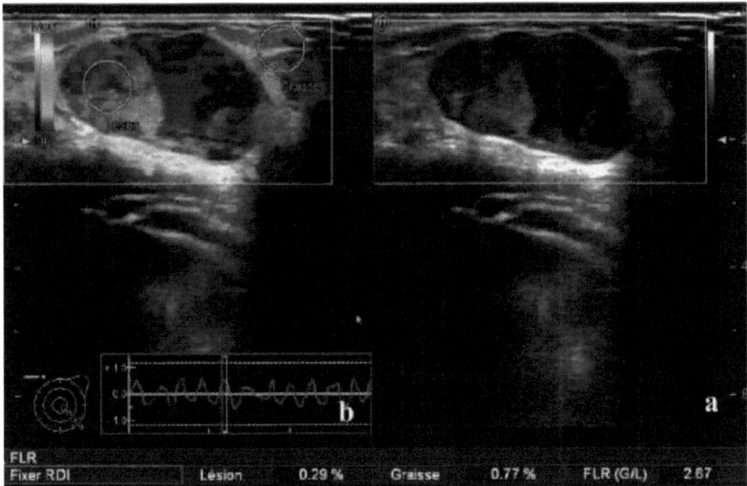

Fig. 81: Intracystic papillary carcinoma in a 73-year-old woman. (a) Ultrasound image. Complex, oval-shaped mass with microlobulated contours and abrupt interface, classified as BI-RADS 4b. (b) Elastographic image. Mass with an elasticity score of 2, a calculated elasticity ratio of 2.67 and a fault ratio of 1.

6.5. Combination of B mode ultrasound and elastographic parameters for lesions classified as BI-RADS 3 and 4a

As a reminder, among the 298 benign masses, short-term follow-up (BI-RADS 3) was recommended in 76 lesions and biopsy (BI-RADS 4a, BI-RADS 4b, BIRADS 4c and BI-RADS 5) was indicated in 222 lesions (table 107).

By following our study protocol, which was to downgrade by one BIRADS category lesions found to be negative in all three elastographic parameters, 79.28% (176/222) of biopsies of benign lesions could have been avoided. However, the number of short-term surveillance of benign lesions (BIRADS 3) increased from 25.5% to 84.56% (table 108).

The majority of masses were classified as BI-RADS 3 and BIRADS 4a (71.47%), including two malignant lesions classified as BI-RADS 4a. None of the two malignant lesions showed negative results for the three elastographic parameters. To this end, we suggested downgrading the masses classified as BI-RADS 3 and 4a which showed negative results for the three elastographic parameters to BI-RADS 2, reducing the short-term follow-up for benign lesions to 98.01% (table 108).

Table 107. Distribution of the results of the B mode ultrasound scanner combination and elastographic parameters.

Category BIRADS	3		4a		4b		4c		5	
Elastographic parameters	**Malin**	**Benin**	**Malin**	**Benin**	**Malin**	**Benin**	**Malin**	**Benin**	**Malin**	**Benin**
All negative	0	71	0	176	1	6	0	20	0	1

parameters										
One or two positive parameters	0	5	2	13	3	1	6	1	1	0
All positive parameters	0	0	0	1	0	0	12	2	52	1
Total	0	76	2	190	4	7	18	23	53	2

Table 108. Management of 77 malignant lesions and 298 benign lesions diagnosed by ultrasound.

Support	**Ultrasound mode B**	**Ultrasound + Elastography**	
Malignant		**Retrograde 4a=>3**	**Retrograde 4a and 3 => 2**
Short-term monitoring	0	0	0
Biopsy	77	77	77
Benign			
Short-term monitoring	76	252 (+176)	5 (- 247)
Biopsy	222	46 (-176)	46 (-176)

6.6. Performance according to histological type

Table 109 shows the results of the combination of B mode ultrasound and elastography according to histological type.

113 fibroadenomas were reclassified as BI-RADS 3. The proportion of fibroadenomas classified as BI-RADS 3 increased from 29.63% to 89.42% thanks to elastography.

23 phyllodes tumours were reclassified as BI-RADS 3. The proportion of phyllodes tumours classified as BI-RADS 3 rose from 6.67% to 83.33%.

32 fibrocystic mastopathy lesions were reclassified as BI-RADS 3. Thanks to elastography, the proportion of fibrocystic mastopathy classified as BIRADS 3 rose from 27.27% to 83.33%.

Two out of four adenomyo-epithelioma lesions were reclassified as BI-RADS 3.

One papilloma in three was reclassified as BI-RADS 3.

Five miscellaneous benign lesions (one PASH lesion, two galactophoritis, one granulomatous mastitis and one reworked cyst) were reclassified as BI-RADS 3. The proportion of miscellaneous benign lesions classified as BI-RADS 3 rose from 17.65% to 47.06%.

All malignant lesions remain classified BI-RADS 4 or 5.

Table 109. Distribution of the results of the combination of B mode ultrasound and elastographic parameters according to histological type.

Histological type	**n = 375**	**US mode B**					**US mode B + Elastography**		
		3	4a	**4b**	**4c**	**5**	**3**	**4/5**	**Reclassify**
Fibroadenoma	189	56	119	2	12	0	169	20	113
Phyllodes tumour	30	2	25	2	1	0	25	5	23
Fibrocystic mastopathy	55	15	35	1	4	0	47	8	32
Adenomyo-epithelioma	4	0	4	0	0	0	2	2	2

Papilloma	**3**	0	1	**0**	2	0	1	2	1
Other benign lesions	17	3	6	2	4	2	8	9	5
CCIS	2	0	0	**0**	2	0	0	2	0
CI NST	55	0	1	3	9	42	0	55	0
CLI	**9**	0	0	**0**	3	6	0	9	0
Mixed carcinoma	4	0	0	**0**	1	3	0	4	0
Other malignant lesions	7	0	1	1	3	2	0	7	0
Total	375	76	192	11	41	55	252	123	176

6.7. Performance as a function of palpability

As shown in Table 110, palpability does not appear to affect specificity (non-palpable masses 84.86% vs palpable masses 83.75%,^ = *0.85).*

Table 110. Diagnostic performance of the ultrasound-elastography combination as a function of palpability.

	Sensitivity	Specific	VPP	VPN	Accuracy
Palpation (-)	**100% [83,89-100]**	**84,86% [79,5-89,01]**	**37,74% [25,94-51,19]**	**100% [97,97-100]**	**86,13% [81,17-89,95]**
Palpation (+)	**100% [93,69-100]**	**83,75% [74,16-90,25]**	**81,43% [70,77-88,81]**	**100% [94,58-100]**	**90,51% [84,44-94,37]**

6.8. Performance as a function of lesion visibility on mammography

Specificity appears to be lower for lesions visible on mammography, but without significant difference (visible lesions 80% vs non-visible lesions 83.49%,^ = *0.58*) (table 111).

Table 111. F he diagnostic performance of the combination ultrasound-elastography in "onction of the mammographically visible nature of a lesion.

	Sensitivity	Specific	VPP	VPN	Accuracy
Mammography (-)	**100% [67,56-100]**	**83,49% [75,4-89,29]**	**30,77% [16,5-49,99]**	**100% [95,95-100]**	**84,62% [76,99-90,04]**
Mammography (+)	**100% [94,73-100]**	**80% [70,86-86,81]**	**78,41% [68,72-85,72]**	**100% [95,19-100]**	**88,41% [82,61-92,46]**

6.9. Performance as a function lesion size

As a reminder, performance as function of size was assessed in relation to the median lesion size, which was 16.5 mm.

Specificity was lower for large lesions (78.03% vs 89.76%, p = *0.006*) (table 112).

Table 112. Diagnostic performance of combined ultrasound-elastography as a function of lesion size.

Distance from skin	Sensitivity	Specific	VPP	VPN	Accuracy
< 16.5 mm	**100% [83,89-100]**	**89,76% [84,21-93,51]**	**54,05% [38,38-68,96]**	**100% [97,49-100]**	**90,86% [85,85-94,22]**
> 16.5 mm	**100% [93,69-100]**	**78,03% [70,23-84,25]**	**66,28% [55,78-75,38]**	**100% [96,4-100]**	**84,66% [78,83-89,1]**

6.10. Performance as a function of skin-to-skin distance lesion

As shown in Table 113, the depth of the lesion does not appear to affect the diagnostic performance of the ultrasound-elastography combination *(p~l)*.

Table 113. Diagnostic performance of combined ultrasound-elastography as a function of skin-to-lesion distance.

Size	Sensitivity	Specificity	VPP	NPV	Accuracy
< 15 mm	100% [95-100]	84,53% [79,68-88,39]	64,04% [54,9-72,25]	100% [98,31-100]	87,87% [83,96-90,93]
> 15 mm	100% [51,01-100]	84,85% [69,08-93,35]	44,44% [18,88-93,35]	100% [87,94-100]	86,49% [72,02-94,09]

CHAPTER 3

Discussion

In this chapter, we will discuss our results and compare them with the literature. We detail diagnostic performance of elastography in the differentiation benign and malignant masses. We then compare the performance of elastography with that of B-mode ultrasound, as well as the performance of the combination of the two examinations. We also discuss diagnostic performance as a function of palpability, mammographic visibility, tumour size and depth. Finally, we will correlate the elastographic results with the histological results.

1. Elastography

1.1. Quality parameters

Elastography was initially based on the colour mapping score proposed by Itoh [84].

In our study, the best threshold value of the elasticity score for differentiation between benign and malignant masses was between score 3 and 4 with a sensitivity of 89.61%, a specificity of 97.65%, a positive predictive value (PPV) of 90.79%, a negative predictive value (NPV) of 97.32% and an accuracy of 96%. Our results are similar to those already described in the literature [49, 84, 126, 133-135, 143, 153-159] (tableaull4).

Itoh et al [84] published one of the first studies to evaluate the diagnostic potential of static elastography on 111 masses, 59 of which were benign and 52 malignant, less than 30 mm in diameter. The elastographic images were classified according to the five scores proposed by the authors. The mean elasticity score was significantly higher in malignant lesions (score 4.2 + 0.9) than in benign lesions (score 2.1 + 1). For a threshold value of between 3 and 4, elastography achieved a sensitivity of 86.5%, a specificity of 89.8% and an accuracy of 88.3%. The results of this study show a good correlation between elastographic scores and histological data.

Giuseppetti et al [139] evaluated the value of static elastography in the study of 91 masses, 27 of which were benign and 64 malignant. This study evaluated the elasticity score proposed by d'Itoh [84]. The sensitivity and specificity of elastography were 79% and 89%, respectively. The authors found that the histological type and size of the lesions influenced the elasticity score.

Between 2006 and 2011, several studies were carried out. A meta-analysis by Gong [153] evaluated 23 articles from 212 references. A threshold value of elasticity score between score 3 and 4 was observed in the different studies. The mean sensitivity was 83.4% (95% CI: 81.4 - 85.3%) with a specificity of 84.2 (95% CI: 82.9 - 85.4%) and an AUC of 0.93.

The study by Stoian et al [154] 174 lesions including 102 benign masses and 72 malignant masses. Scores 1, 2 and 3 were considered as benign lesions and scores 4 and 5 as malignant. The authors found a sensitivity of 82.9%, a specificity of 81.9%, a PPV of 80.3%, a NPV of 82.2%, and an accuracy of 96%.

The recent study by Khamis [155], which evaluated the elasticity score of 120 masses (75 benign and 45 malignant), found a sensitivity of 100%, a specificity of 88%, a PPV of 83.3%, a NPV of 100%, an accuracy of 92.5% and an AUC of 0.98.

In our study, of the 8 false-negatives, three were infiltrating NST carcinomas, one cribriform carcinoma, one micro-papillary cancer, one papillary intracystic cancer, one mucinous carcinoma and one ductal carcinoma in situ. These data are consistent with the literature.

In the study by Houelleu Demay et al [160], of the 12 false negatives, six were infiltrating NST carcinomas, two infiltrating lobular carcinomas, one mucinous-type carcinoma and one ductal carcinoma in situ.

In the series by Tardivon et al. 61 malignant lesions and 61 benign lesions, the histology of the 13 false-negatives (scores 1, 2 and 3) corresponded to infiltrating NST carcinomas in 8 cases, infiltrating lobular carcinomas in three cases, one colloid type cancer and one papillary cancer [92].

In the series by Giuseppetti et al (91 masses), the histology of 13 false-negatives (elastographic scores of 2 and 3) corresponded to infiltrating carcinomas of the mixed type (n = 6), infiltrating lobular carcinomas (n = 3) and infiltrating carcinomas of the NST type (n = 4) [139].

Among our 8 elastographic false-negatives, there was a mucinous cancer with a gelatinous consistency due to abundant mucus secretion. There was also a lobular cancer and an in situ cancer for which a benign colorimetric score is explained by the fact that in these three first lesions, there is no desmoplastic fibrous reaction.

Our study shows a good correlation between elastographic scores and the hardness of the tissue studied, which is the very principle of this technique. In fact, false-positive elastography was found in lesions with hard or fibrous structures that gave rise to a high pejorative score (granulomatous mastitis, cytosteatonecrosis, fibroadenoma) and may involve partially calcified lesions.

Table 114. Diagnostic performance of the elasticity score according to published series.

Authors	Number	Sensitivity	Specific	VPP	VPN	Accuracy
Itoh [84] 2006	111	86.5%	89.8%	NP	NP	88.3%
Zhu [121] 2008	139	88,5%%	88,6%	NP	NP	87%
Raza [126] 2010	128	92,7%	85,8%	76%	96%	88,3%
Regini [134] 2010	120	88.5%	92,7%	86,1%	94,1%	91,3%
Schaefer [133] 2011	193	96,9%	76%	NP	NP	NP
Gong [153] 2011	128	95%	93,9%	76,5%	73,7%	94,7%
Navarro [156] 2011	124	69.5%	83.1%	78.9%	75.0%	NP
Yerli [141] 2011	78	80%	95%	84%	93%	91%
Stachs[135] 2013	224	87,9%	73,1%	77,9%	84,9%	80,9%
Stoian [154] 2016	174	82,9%	81,9%	80,3%	83,9%	82,2%
Menezes [157] 2016	100	100%	82,7%	65,8%	100%	87%

Arslan [158] 2017	81	71,1%	97,7%	96,4%	79,2%	85,1%
Bojanic [159] 2017	117	90,5%	93%	86%	95%	92,5%
Khamis [155] 2017	120	100%	88%	83,3%	100%	92,5%
Our study	375	89,61%	97,65%	90,79%	97,32%	96%
NP: Not specified						

1.2. Quantitative parameters

1.2.1. Semi-quantitative analysis

In elastography, Itoh et al [84] suggested five elasticity scores, after which this was widely used to distinguish between malignant and benign masses [144, 159]. On the other hand, many subjective factors can alter the elastographic score of lesions. In practice, it is sometimes difficult to differentiate between scores 2 and 3 on the elastographic image [97]. Consequently, the development of a new method that could reduce this bias as much as possible is necessary [87].

The elasticity ratio, a more objective method than the elasticity score, has been used to discriminate semi-quantitatively the hardness of breast lesions. It is a simple, practical method that is easy to learn [144, 161, 162].

1.2.1.1. FLRouGLR

In our study, we performed two measures of elasticity ratio, the *Fat-Lesion* Ratio (FLR) and the *Gland-Lesion Ratio* (GLR). Our results showed that both the FLR and GLR of malignant lesions were significantly higher than those of benign lesions *($p<0.0001$ for both).*

The FLR had a sensitivity of 96.1% and a specificity of 93.3% in the diagnosis of breast lesions, while the GLR offered a sensitivity of 72% and a specificity of 81.1% (table 115).

Comparison of the two ratios showed that the FLR had a better diagnostic performance than the GLR (AUC, 0.990 vs 0.820,j9 < *0.0001).*

Subcutaneous fat was considered the most appropriate structure for calculating the elasticity ratio as it is not influenced by other factors such as breast density, hormonal status, menstrual cycle and lactation [85, 86, 96, 140, 163]. According to Jung et al [164], FLR values were not influenced by the position of the ROI in the reference fat tissue whatever the depth of the lesion.

Previous studies have shown that glandular tissue and adipose tissue have different elasticity. In an in vitro study, Krouskop et al [73] found that the elastic modulus of glandular tissue was significantly higher than that of adipose tissue. In an in vivo study using shear wave elastography, Zhou et al [165] reported that glandular tissue was harder than fatty tissue in both benign and malignant groups.

In the study published by Zhou et al [166] the lesion/fatty tissue ratio (with a cut-off value of 2.78) had a sensitivity of 82.9% and a specificity of 75.6%, while the lesion/glandular tissue ratio (with a cut-off value of 1.54) had a sensitivity of 77.1% and a specificity of 69.9%.

In the study by Graziano et al [167], the FLR (cut-off value of 3) had a sensitivity of 71.1% and a specificity of 75%, results that were slightly better than those of the GLR, which for a cut-off value of 2.15 had a sensitivity of 83% and a specificity of 70.8%; however, this difference was not significant.

Table 115. Diagnostic performance of the FLR and GLR elasticity ratios.

Authors	n	Parameters	Threshold value	Sensitivity	Specific
Zhou [166] 2014	193	FLR	3,91	82,9%	75,6%
		GLR	2,15	77,5%	69,9%
Graziano [167] 2017	159	FLR	3,00	71,7%	75,0%
		GLR	2,15	83,0%	70,8%
Our study	375	FLR	3,67	96,1%	93,3%
		GLR	1,87	72.0%	81,1%.

1.2.1.2. Elasticity ratio

In general, benign breast lesions had a lower elasticity ratio than malignant lesions. mean elasticity ratio of benign lesions in our study was 2.10 + 1.18, which was significantly lower than the mean elasticity ratio of malignant lesions (32.74 ± 39.86), in agreement with other studies [85-87, 154-157, 159, 168-172] (Table 116).

Zhao et al [144] noted that the mean elasticity ratio was 2.06 ± 1.27 for benign lesions and 6.66 ± 4.62 for malignant lesions, with a high significant difference. Similarly, in the study by Menezes et al [157], the mean elasticity ratio of benign lesions was 3.87 ± 3.52, significantly lower than that of malignant lesions (8.99 ± 5.34).

Determining a universal elasticity ratio cut-off value to differentiate benign from malignant masses is one of the major challenges in the practice of elastography. Several previously published studies have determined an elasticity ratio cut-off value for better differentiation of benign and malignant lesions but these studies had different cut-off values [85-87, 154-157, 158, 168-172].

Zhi et al [87] found that the best threshold value at which malignant and benign lesions could be accurately identified was 3.05 with a sensitivity of 92.4% and a specificity of 91.1%.

Similarly, Mu et al [173] found that at a threshold value of 3.01, the elasticity ratio had a sensitivity of 79.8% and a specificity of 82.8%.

Studies were carried out in 2010-2011. In this respect, a meta-analysis by Sadigh [123] evaluated 12 articles from 3000 references. The threshold elasticity ratio for differentiating malignant from benign tumours varied between 0.5 and 4.5. The mean sensitivity was 88%, with a specificity of 83%.

In our study, the threshold value was set at 3.67, with a sensitivity of 96.1% and a specificity of 93.3%. Gheoneaet al [174] observed a sensitivity of 93.3% and a specificity of 92.9%, for a cut-off value equivalent to that in our study (3.67). A higher cut-off value of 3.77 was reported by Khamis et al [155] with a sensitivity of 93.3% and a specificity of 97.3%.

Despite significant differences between malignant and benign lesions observed on elastography, some lesions had misleading elastographic characteristics. For example, for three malignant lesions the values of the elasticity ratio were in favour of benignity; they were below the threshold value of 3.67. All the false negatives in our study corresponded to an infiltrating NST carcinoma, a micro-papillary carcinoma and an intracystic papillary carcinoma.

Tardivon et al [92] also showed that false negatives on elastography were generally ductal carcinomas in situ or invasive carcinomas without a desmoplastic reaction [175, 176]. Other studies have shown that lobular carcinomas or NST, mucinous carcinomas or ductal carcinomas in situ can also give rise to false-negative cases on elastography [92, 160], with no histological specificity demonstrated [84].

In our study, 20 benign lesions had elasticity ratio values in favour of malignancy, i.e. above the threshold value of 3.67. These false-positive elastographs corresponded to particular benign lesions (fibrocystic mastopathies, adenomyo-epithelioma, papilloma, epidermal cyst) or with histological characteristics that could explain their hardness (phyllodes tumours, fibroadenomas, cytosteatonecrosis, granulomatous mastitis). In the majority of cases, imaging in B mode was also suspicious (11 BI-RADS 4 lesions, one BI-RADS 5 lesion) and did not allow biopsy to be deferred.

A study by Thomas et al [86] suggested that a lower threshold value for the elasticity ratio (2.45) could improve the sensitivity of this method, thereby reducing the number of false-negative results. To correctly identify all breast cancers in our study, a threshold elasticity ratio of less than 2.66 would be required to achieve 100% sensitivity and 83.8% specificity. To achieve 100% specificity, a threshold elasticity ratio of more than 5.94 would be required, with a sensitivity of 86%.

Table 6. Diagnostic performance of the elasticity ratio according to published series.

Authors	n	Threshold value	Sensitivity	Specific	VPP	VPN	Accuracy
Thomas [86] 2010	227	2,45	90%	88%	88,8%	90%	89,4%
Kumm [177] 2010	310	2,45	79%	76%	57%	90%	77%
Zhi [87] 2010	559	3,05	92,4%	91,1%	78,2%	97,2%	91,4%
Lee [142]2011	315	2	68,8%%	64,8%	26%	92%	NP
Yerli [141] 2011	78	3.52	80%	93%	80%	93%	90%
Cho [96] 2011	99	2,24	95%	75%	48,7%	98,3%	78,8%
Farrokh [85] 2011	117	2,9	92,6%	95,2%	94,3%	93,7%	94%
Gheonea [174] 2011	58	3,67	93,3%	92,9%	NP	NP	NP
Stachs[135] 2013	224	2	90,70%	58,2%	70,3%	88,1%	75,1%
Stoian [154] 2016	175	4,88	86,5%	90,4%	88,9%	88,2%	88,5%
Menezes [157] 2016	100	4,72	92%	74,6%	NP	NP	NP
Redling [168] 2016	164	2,5	57%	83%	68%	75%	NP
Balçik [169] 2016	135	4,52	85,5%	84,8%	85,5%	84,8%	85,2%
Seo [171]2017	45	2,63	95%	88%	NP	NP	NP
Bojanic [159] 2017	117	3,5	87,5%	87,6%	75,5%	93,8%	89,9%

Arslan [158] 2017	81	2,84	78,9%	90,7%	88,2%	82,9%	85,1%
Khamis [155] 2017	120	3,77	93,3%	97,3%	95,5%	96,1%	95,8%
Zhao [172] 2018	1071	2,98	86,9%	86,6%	NP	NP	NP
Dawood [170] 2018	40	3	96,7%	100%	NP	NP	NP
Our study	375	3,67	96,1%	93,29%	78,72%	98,93%	93,87%
NP: Not specified							

1.2.2. Size ratio

An important feature of malignant tumours, which appear larger on the elastographic image than on B-mode ultrasound [178-180]. This may result from local infiltration of cancer cells that is not always evident on B-mode ultrasound.

In our series, malignant lesions had a higher size ratio than benign lesions. The mean size ratio of malignant lesions was 1.23 + 0.22, significantly higher than that of benign lesions, 0.99 + 0.05 *($p < 0.0001$)*, in agreement with other studies [89, 65, 157] (table 117).

Menezes et al [157] found that the mean size ratio for malignant lesions was 1.13 ± 0.36 and 1.02 ± 0.25 for benign lesions with a high significant difference *($p < 0.0001$)*. Also, in the study by Leong et al [65] the mean size ratio of malignant lesions was significantly higher than that of benign lesions (1.75 ± 0.72 vs 1.04 ± 0.39,j9 < *0.0001)*.

Barr et al [142], in a multicentre study including 222 malignant lesions and 431 benign lesions, demonstrated that benign and malignant lesions can be distinguished by size ratio. A size ratio greater than 1 was found in 219 malignant lesions out of 222, and a size ratio less than 1 was found in 361 benign lesions out of 431, giving a sensitivity of 98.6% and a specificity of 87.4%.

Our study, for a size ratio cut-off value of 1.045, showed a sensitivity of 87.01%, a specificity of 93.29%, a PPV of 91.78%, a NPV of 96.69% and an accuracy of 95.73%.

Barr et al [89] presented similar results to our study. In another series of 251 lesions, 197 were benign and 54 malignant. Of the 54 malignant lesions, all had a size ratio equal to or greater than 1. Of the 197 benign lesions, 187 had a size ratio less than 1 and 10 benign lesions had a size ratio greater than 1. The authors found a sensitivity of 100%, a specificity of 95%, a PPV of 84%, a NPV of 100% and an accuracy of 96%.

Leong et al [65], for a size ratio threshold value of 1.1, found a sensitivity of 92%, a specificity of 69%, a PPV of 48%, a NPV of 96.7% and an accuracy of 74.5%.

In our study, of ten false-negative size ratios, five were infiltrating NST carcinomas, one cribriform carcinoma, one papillary intracystic carcinoma, one colloid carcinoma and two intracanal carcinomas.

Among the 10 elastographic false negatives found, one colloid type cancer, one papillary intracystic cancer and two in situ cancers for which the size ratio was below the threshold value is explained by the fact that in these first four lesions, there is no desmoplastic fibrous reaction.

Of the 5 false negatives corresponding to infiltrating NST carcinomas, four were grade II and III, rapidly progressive, and did not develop stromal reaction [175, 176].

The false positives in our study included three cases of granulomatous mastitis, one cytosteatonecrosis lesion, one abscess and one adenomyo-epithelioma.

Of these 6 false positives, 5 lesions were of inflamammatous origin (3 granulomatous mastitis, cytosteatonecrosis, abscess) in which a peripheral inflamammatous infiltrate rich in macrophages and giant cells is organised, subsequently progressing to fibrosis, which explains the high size ratio values.

Table 117. Diagnostic performance of the size ratio according to published series.

Authors	n	Threshold value	Sensitivity	Specific	VPP	VPN	Accuracy
Leong [65] 2010	110	1,1	92%	69%	48%	96,7%	74,5%
Barr [89] 2010	251	1	100%	95%	84,4%	100%	96%
Menezes [157] 2016	100	1,19	84%	85,33%	NP	NP	NP
Our study	375	1,045	87,01%	97,99%	91,78 %	96,69 %	95,73%

NP: Not specified

1.3. Comparison of the performance of elastographic parameters

The results of our study showed that the elasticity score, the elasticity ratio and the size ratio have excellent diagnostic performances in the differentiation of benign and malignant masses. The AUC value was 0.936 for the elasticity score, 0.947 for the elasticity ratio and 0.925 for the size ratio. The sensitivity, specificity, PPV, NPV and accuracy of the elasticity score were 89.61%, 97.65%, 90.79% 97.32% and 96% respectively, for the elasticity ratio the values were 96.1%, 93.29%, 78.72%, 98.93% and 93.87% respectively and for the size ratio they were 87.01%, 97.99%, 91.78%, 96.69% and 95.73% respectively. However, there was no significant difference between the three methods.

Khamis et al [155] also found high diagnostic performance for the elasticity score and ratio, with no significant difference between the two methods. The sensitivity, specificity, PPV, NPV and accuracy of the elasticity score were 100%, 88%, 83.3%, 100% and 92.5% respectively, and for the elasticity ratio they were 93.3%, 97.3%, 95.5%, 96.1% and 95.8% respectively.

Mutala [181] compared the diagnostic performance of the score and the elasticity ratio and concluded that the elasticity ratio was highly accurate in differentiating benign and malignant masses, but there was no significant difference between the two parameters.

Despite the fact that the elastographic parameters have comparable diagnostic performances, calculation of the elasticity ratio seems to be mandatory, particularly for large masses and to differentiate between elasticity scores 3 and 4 [173].

In contrast, the study by Jung [164] evaluated the size ratio, the elasticity ratio and the elasticity score and concluded that the elasticity ratio showed the best diagnostic performance of the three elastographic parameters.

Menezes et al [157] compared 4 elastographic parameters, namely the elasticity score, the elasticity ratio, the size ratio and the surface area ratio. They demonstrated that the elasticity score had the best diagnostic performance of the 4 parameters.

Yerli et al. presented a study of 78 lesions to determine whether the combination of elasticity score and elasticity ratio was useful in differentiating benign from malignant lesions [141]. They concluded that after evaluation by the elastography elasticity score, the additional use of the elasticity ratio did not contribute to the differentiation between benign and malignant lesions.

2. Diagnostic performance of elastography and ultrasound mode B

In our study, B-mode ultrasound had a higher sensitivity than elastography (100% vs 89.*61%,p = 0.01*). On the other hand, elastography had a higher specificity than B-mode ultrasound (97.65% vs 25.5%,j9 < *0.0001).* These results are in agreement with previous studies [68, 157, 158] in which elastography showed better specificity (ranged from 82.7% to 98.5%) than B-mode ultrasound (ranged from 7.1% to 87.1%) (table 117).

The study by Itoh et al [84], involving 111 lesions, found a sensitivity of 96.2% and a specificity of 62.7% for mode B ultrasound. On the other hand, for elastography with a threshold value between scores 3 and 4, they found a sensitivity of 86.5% and a specificity of 89.8%.

Arslan et al [158] compared elastography with B-mode ultrasound. 81 lesions were studied. Elastography had a higher specificity than B-mode ultrasound (90.7% vs ll.6%,j9 < *0.0001*). Whereas sensitivity was lower than that of B-mode ultrasound (100% vs 78.9%,*p < 0.0001).*

Zhi et al [87] compared elastography and B-mode ultrasound in the differentiation of benign and malignant breast lesions. They studied 401 lesions (246 benign, 155 malignant) using the elasticity score devised by Itoh et al [84]. Elastography had a higher specificity than B-mode ultrasound (91.9% vs 68.3%, p < 0.0001). Diagnostic accuracy and PPV were higher than B-mode ultrasound, 84.4% vs 76.8% and 86.2% vs 64.2%, respectively. Whereas sensitivity, NPV were lower than those of B-mode ultrasound (90.3% vs 72.3% and 91.8% vs 84.1%, respectively).

Balçik et al [169], in a study of 135 lesions, observed a sensitivity of 98.5% and a specificity of 56.2% for mode B ultrasound. On the other hand, for elastography with a threshold value between scores 3 and 4, they found a sensitivity of 80% and a specificity of 90.8%.

Table 118. Diagnostic performance of the elasticity score according to published series.

Authors	η	Technical	Sensitivity	Specific	VPP	VPN
Itoh [84] 2006	111	US Mode B	92,2%	62,7%	NP	NP
		USE	86,5%	89,8%	NP	NP
Zhi [87] 2010	401	US Mode B	90,3%	68,3%	64,2%	91,8%

		USE	73,3%	91,9%	86,2%	91,2%
Tardivon [92] 2007	122	US Mode B	98,4%	47,5%	65,2%	96,9%
		USE	78,7%	86,9%	85,7%	80,3%
Raza [126] 2010	188	US Mode B	100%	7,1%	34,1%	100%
		USE	83,6%	87,4%	76,15	91,7%
Thomas [98] 2006	108	US Mode B	91,8%	78%	NP	NP
		USE	77,6%	91,5%	NP	NP
Zhu [121] 2008	139	US Mode B	94,2%	87,1%	NP	NP
		USE	85,5%	88,6%	NP	NP
Hatzung [182] 2010	97	US Mode B	97%	82%	71%	98%
		USE	71%	89%	79%	92%
Yerli [141] 2011	78	US Mode B	87,5%	72,6%	45,2%	95,7%
		USE	80%	95%	84%	93%
Redling [168] 2016	164	US Mode B	95%	81%	76%	96%
		USE	39%	94%	82%	71%
Balçik [169] 2016	135	US Mode B	98,5%	56,2%	71,1%	97,2%
		USE	80%	90,8%	90,3%	80,8%
Menezes [157] 2016	100	US Mode B	100%	70,66%	53,19%	100%
		USE	100%	82,7%	65,8%	100%
Areslan [158] 2017	81	US Mode B	100%	11,6%	50%	100%
		USE	71,1%	97,7%	96,4%	79,2%
Our study	375	US Mode B	100 %	25,5 %	25,75%	100 %
		USE	89,61%	97,7%	90,8%	97,32%

NP: Not specified

3. Diagnostic performance of combinations of B-mode ultrasound with different elastographic parameters.

The BI-RADS lexicon is a system for classifying ultrasound images according to their morphological characteristics [10]. This classification system only describes the morphological characteristics of lesions with high sensitivity values, but the specificity values of ultrasound BI-RADS are still below the desired level.

Elastography can be used in combination with B-mode ultrasound to improve diagnostic performance. Thus, in addition to the morphological character obtained by BI-RADS, elastography can inform us, about the hardness of the lesions [183].

Hao et al [184] combined the elasticity score with the BI-RADS classification. they showed an improvement in specificity from 48.7% to 82.1%, PPV from 56.1% to 77.8% and accuracy from 68.8% to 77.8%.

In another study by Zhi et al [185], the authors combined B-mode ultrasound with elastography and showed that elastography improved the specificity, PPV and accuracy of B-mode ultrasound alone from 68.3% to 87.8%, from 64.2% to 76.5% and from 76.8% to 86.3%, respectively.

In a multicentre study by Lee et al [186], the authors evaluated the combination of B mode ultrasound with elastography as part of screening in women with dense breasts, noting that the combination reduced the false positive rate and consequently improved specificity from 27% to 74% and PPV from 8.9% to 20.3%.

Arslan et al [158] separately combined the elasticity score and elasticity ratio with B-mode ultrasound and concluded that the combination of qualitative or quantitative elastography improved the diagnostic performance of B-mode ultrasound alone. The combination of ultrasound and elasticity score improved specificity from 11.6% to 97.7%, PPV from 50% to 97.1% and accuracy from 53% to 92.5%.

In addition, the ultrasound-elasticity ratio combination increased the specificity, PPV and accuracy of B-mode ultrasound, respectively, by
11.6% to 93%, 50% to 91.9% and 53% to 91.3%.

Our study is in agreement with the results in the literature. The combined use of the elasticity score with B-mode ultrasound significantly improved AUC from 0.628 to 0.936, specificity from 25.5% to 97.65%, PPV from 25.75% to 90.79% and accuracy from 40.8% to 96% (allj9 < *0.0001*). By adding the elasticity ratio to the elasticity score-B-mode ultrasound combination, this combination increased specificity and PPV to 98.32% and 90.79% respectively.

Comparing the diagnostic performance of the different combinations of mode B ultrasound with the qualitative and quantitative parameters of elastography, the combination of the three parameters of elastography with mode B ultrasound revealed a very high diagnostic performance with a specificity of 98.66% and a PPV of 94.12% compared with the other combinations and mode B ultrasound alone.

However, thanks to our method combining B-mode ultrasound with the qualitative and quantitative parameters of elastography, the number of false positives would be reduced from 222 to 4.

In our study, 190 of the 192 masses classified as BI-RADS 4a could be downgraded to BI-RADS 3 if they showed negative results for the three elastographic parameters. The number of lesions correctly downgraded to BI-RADS 3 would be 176 out of 190, i.e. 92.63% of lesions classified as BI-RADS 4a. This could reduce the number of false positives and consequently the number of unnecessary biopsies, which represented 79.28% (176/222) of the biopsies performed in our study. Our results are in agreement with those in the literature [184, 185, 187, 188].

Cho's study [189] reported that 44% of biopsies of benign lesions classified as BI-RADS 4a and scored let 2 could have been avoided.

Yi et al [187] reported that 38.2% (485 out of 1269) of biopsies of benign lesions were useless.

In our series, no malignant lesion was downgraded to BI-RADS 3. To this end, we suggested that masses classified as BI-RADS 3 and 4a which showed negative results for the three elastographic parameters should be downgraded to BIRADS 2. We reduced the short-term surveillance recommended for benign lesions by

98.01%. Our study is similar to that of Lee et al.
[186] who showed that the combined use of B mode ultrasound and elastography reduced the number of unnecessary biopsies by 57.76% for benign lesions and short-term follow-up by 89.32%.

4. Performance as a function of palpability

In our study, palpability did not affect the specificity of elastography (non-palpable masses 84.86% vs palpable masses 83.75%,j9 = *0.85*). This corroborates the study by Yoon et al [143], who reported that there was no significant difference between concordant and discordant elastographic images of palpable and non-palpable lesions ($p > 0.05$).

5. Performance as a function of lesion visibility on mammography

are very few studies in the literature on the three imaging , mammography, ultrasound and elastography [93, 190, 191].

In our study, we observed that lesion hardness was correlated with the visibility of lesions on mammography ($p < 0.0001$) and that the specificity of the ultrasound-elastography combination was not affected by the visibility of lesions on mammography ($p = 0.58$).

Mohey et al [190] found that the sensitivity of mammography alone (72.7%) was greater than that of ultrasonography in mode B (69.7%) or elastography (69.7%). The specificity of elastography (95.1%) was greater than that of mammography (86.4%) and ultrasound (72.8%). The ultrasound-elastography combination obtained the best results for cancer detection (sensitivity of 90.9%, specificity of 95.1% and accuracy of 93.8%).

6. Performance as a function lesion size

In our study, specificity was lower for larger lesions (78.03% vs 89.76%,^ = *0.006).*

Our study is in agreement with Liu et al [192], who reported that when tumour size is small, the difference in hardness between benign lesions and breast tissue is small and consequently the score and elasticity ratio values are low.

Most small malignant lesions do not contain internal necrosis and the hardness of the lesions is relatively homogeneous. As a result, the false negative rate is lower with elastography. In large lesions, calcifications, fibrosis and necrosis may be present, possibly resulting in uneven hardness, which is responsible for false negatives [193, 194].

7. Performance as a function of depth

The depth of the lesion does not appear to affect the diagnostic performance of the ultrasound-elastography combination *(p~l).*

Yoon et al [143] found no significant difference between lesion depth and elastography performance.

Carlsen et al [195] evaluated the elasticity scores of targets of different depths using static elastography and shear wave elastography and observed that the AUC of static elastography was higher than that of shear wave elastography and that depth only influences shear wave velocity. Since mass depth does not affect static elastography, it is potentially advantageous over shear wave elastography in the diagnosis of breast masses.

8. Correlations between histological results and elastographic parameters

8.1. Histological type

8.1.1. Benign lesions

In fibro-epithelial tumours, fibroadenomas showed significantly lower values of elasticity ratio than phyllodes (1.97 + 1.14 vs 2.54 + 0.83,j9 = *0.001*), indicating that fibroadenomas are less hard than phyllodes. These results are in agreement with the study by Li et al. where the mean elasticity ratio for fibroadenomas was 1.69 + 0.88 and for phyllodes tumours was 3.19 ± 2.33, $p < 0.001$. What was also found by Kim et al. in shear wave elastography, the mean elasticity of fibroadenomas and phyllodes tumours were respectively 15.8 kPa vs 66.7 kPa, $p < 0.01$ [196, 197]. Phyllodes tumours are histologically characterised by a more abundant and cellular stroma than fibroadenomas [151,198]. Consequently, phyllodes tumours tend to be harder than fibroadenomas.

With regard to histological groups, according to the amount of stremal cellularity, our results showed that moderately cellular fibroadenomas were harder than poorly cellular fibroadenomas, the more stremal cellularity was increased the higher the elasticity ratio was (poorly cellular = 1.88 + 1.15, moderately cellular = 2.33 + 1.03 and highly cellular = 2.53 + 0.83,j9 = *0.002*). Some fibroadenomas with low stremal cellularity tend to be hard on elastography, which may be related to the presence of high levels of stremal fibrosis and calcifications (fig. 82). The reason why the value of the correlation coefficient was moderate may be related to the lack of sensitivity of elastography to clearly reflect the amount of stremal cellularity.

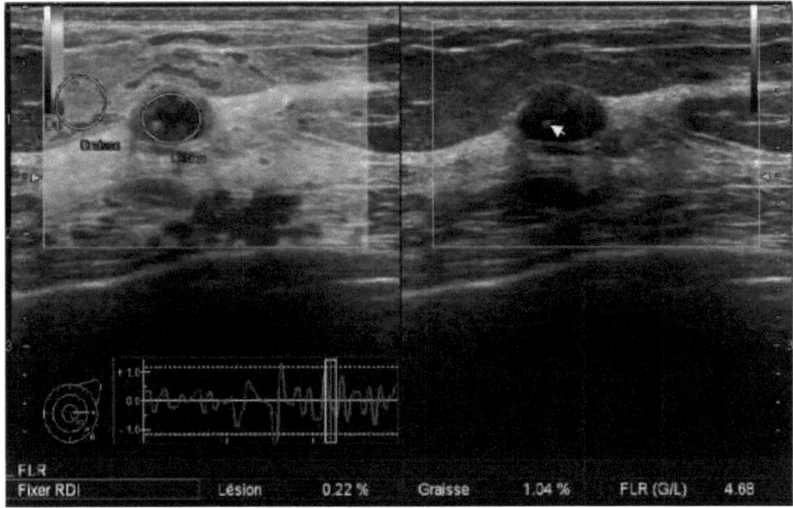

Fig. 82: Low cellularity adenofibroma in a 61-year-old woman. Elastography image. Mass with calcifications (arrow), hard on elastography with a calculated elasticity ratio of 4.68.

8.1.2. Malignant lesions

8.1.2.1. Carcinoma in situ versus invasive carcinoma

A number of previous studies have shown that invasive carcinomas tend to be harder than carcinomas in situ [199-205].

Bae JS et al [202] compared 70 ductal carcinomas in situ against 50 infiltrating NST carcinomas and found higher elasticity values for infiltrating NST carcinomas than for ductal carcinomas in situ, respectively 118.71 ± 70.5 kPa vs 74.8 ± 47.4 kPa$_{5j}$p < *0.0001.*

More recently, Shin J et al [201] also reported higher elasticity values in infiltrating NST carcinomas than in ductal carcinomas in situ (119.04 ± 73.32 kPa vs 85.33 ± 66.1 kPa$_{5j}$p = *0.041).*

This is in agreement with our study, in which the mean elasticity ratio for infiltrating carcinomas was 33.30 + 40.24 and 12.02 + 4.58 for carcinomas in situ *($p < 0.0001$).*

The hardness of infiltrating carcinomas is high. This is partly due to the extracellular fibrous matrix produced by the fibroblasts. Initially, the extracellular matrix was considered to be a passive supporting structure, but it is far from being a structure that only serves to anchor cells. It is capable of playing an active role by sending signals to y resident cells and modulating their behaviour by activating signalling cascades via adhesion receptors or by modulating access to certain molecules of which it is composed [206]. The influence of the extracellular matrix on epithelial cells is not exerted solely through signalling molecules. Indeed, the work of Weaver et al [207] shows that the more rigid the matrix, the greater the increase in epithelial cell growth, alteration of adhesion proteins and loss of polarity. Fibrosis associated with cancer is high in invasive and metastatic cancers [208-211] (fig. 83).

Hao et al [212] prospectively studied the elasticity score of 300 breast lesions, 185 of which were malignant and 115 benign, by correlating the percentage of expression of the a-SMA (Alpha Smooth Muscle Actin) antigen in myofibroblast cells using immunohistochemistry. They described a positive correlation between α-SMA antigen expression and elasticity score (r = 0.487, *p < 0.0001).*

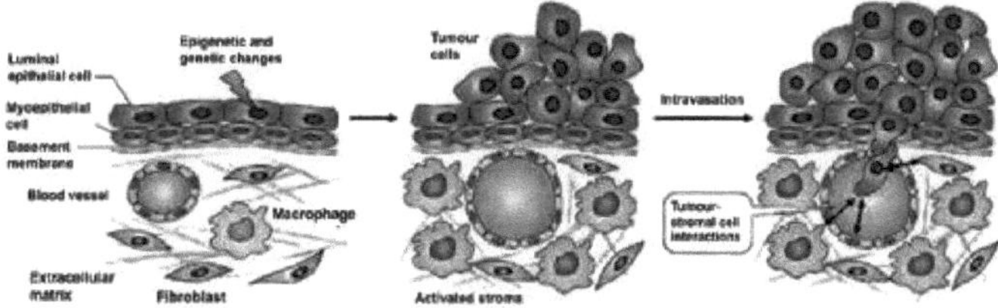

Fig. 83. Classical representation of the tumour stroma. Initially composed of various cell types such as macrophages, fibroblasts and blood vessels, the stroma undergoes major changes as the tumour progresses. The fibroblasts become more active, becoming myofibroblasts, and the number of macrophages increases, leading to increased secretion of growth factors, extracellular matrix components and metalloproteinases [213].

8.1.2.2. Histological types

In our study, lobular carcinomas were harder than other histological types with a mean elasticity ratio of 53.40 + 51.81 vs infiltrating carcinomasNST of 34.55 + 40.43, but without significant difference *(p = 0.16).* Several studies have found no difference in elastography between infiltrating lobular carcinomas and other types of breast cancer [200, 214, 215].

Jin Y et al [214] gave a mean elasticity value for infiltrating lobular carcinomas of 66.12 ± 25.78 compared with a mean elasticity ratio of 82.54 ± 15.64 for infiltrating NST carcinomas *(p = 0.13).*

In the study by Vinnicombe SJ [215], 96.30% of infiltrating lobular carcinomas and 94.32% of infiltrating NST carcinomas had elasticity values greater than 50 kPa *(p = 0.61).*

However, two studies report higher hardness in elastography for infiltrating lobular carcinomas than for non-specific infiltrating cancers. Brkljacié et al [216], compared 75 infiltrating NST carcinomas and 40 infiltrating lobular , the infiltrating lobular carcinomas had a higher mean elasticity than the infiltrating NST carcinomas, respectively 180.41 + 27.06 kPa vs 162.20 + 37.46 kPa,j9 < *0.05.* Similarly, Evans et al [217] reported significantly higher elasticity for infiltrating lobular carcinomas than for infiltrating NST carcinomas, respectively 181 + 67 kPa vs 139 + 56 kPa, *(p < 0.0001).*

Overall, the results reported in the literature vary. In any case, elastography seems to be a particularly interesting tool for increasing the sensitivity of ultrasound for the detection of infiltrating lobular carcinomas, sometimes highlighting areas of suspicious hardness even when there is no clearly identifiable abnormality on B

mode ultrasound [218].
In our series, lobular carcinomas had the highest size ratio values compared with the other histological types *($p < 0.0001$)*. These results are consistent with the study by Grajo JR et al [219] which found a size ratio for infiltrating lobular carcinomas of 1.8 + 0.3 compared with that for infiltrating NST carcinomas of 1.5 + 0.07 ($p < 0.0001$). These results also corroborate the particular histological characteristics of infiltrating lobular carcinomas, which are made up of small, round, non-cohesive cells, isolated or in "Indian file", tending to infiltrate the adjacent breast tissue, without destroying the anatomical structures or causing a frank desmoplastic reaction [220]. This suggests that elastography is a better reflection of the extent of the lesions.

8.1.3. Histopronostic grade

In our series, Grade III tumours were significantly associated with the highest elasticity ratio values (mean elasticity ratio, Grade I of 10.12 ± 5.44, Grade U of 33.10 ± 36.55, Grade Ш of 55.03 ± 62.18,p = *0.017).*
There are controversial results regarding the correlation between histological grade and elastography. Although some found that low grade tumours have the highest elasticity values.
In a series of 291 invasive cancers, Jin Y et al [214] found high elasticity ratio values correlated with low histological grades (Grade 1: 88.58 ± 13.79, Grade II: 87.80 ± 9.90, Grade III: 65.68 ± 18.02,p < *0.0001).*
Similarly Durhan G et al [221] also correlated high histological grade with the lowest values of elasticity ratio (Grade 1: 20.56 ±4.1, Grade II: 23.7 ± 5.7, Grade III: 11.7 ± 5.1; Grade Ш-П,ρ= *0.01* ■ Grade Ш-I,ρ= *0.2).*
On the other hand, in the study by Evans et al, the authors found that grade III was significantly associated with the highest values of hardness (143 kPa median value). The difference in hardness was more marked between grades I and II (85 and 139 kPa respectively) than between grades II and III [217].
Chang et al. in a series of 337 invasive cancers also found a correlation between high tumour grade and high elasticity values (Grade 1: 117.2 ± 53 kPa, Grade II: 132 ± 57.7 kPa, Grade III: 165 ± 52.4 kPa; $p< 0.0001$) [222].
Grajo JR et al. showed that NST grade III infiltrating carcinomas had higher elasticity ratio values than NST grade IandII ($p<0.0001$) [219].
In vitro biophysical studies have shown that tumour hardness is associated with tumour proliferation [223-226].
According to Lee et al, grade III tumours were harder, due to their greater tumour cellularity [227].
Further studies are needed to resolve these discrepancies.

8.1.4. Hormone receptors

The presence of hormone receptors has a good prognosis and indicates that a tumour is hormone-sensitive. Their absence has a poorer prognosis; receptor-negative tumours respond better to chemotherapy.

In our study, hormone receptor-negative tumours were harder than receptor-positive tumours (restrogen receptor, $p = 0.001$ *and* progesterone receptor, $p = 0.007$).

Chang et al. studied the hardness of invasive cancers retrospectively using elastography and correlating receptor status, and found a significant association between mean elasticity and estrogen receptor negativity (mean elasticity of 167 kPa for receptor-negative cancers and 138.7 kPa for receptor-positive cancers, j9 < *0.015*), while the correlation was not significant for progesterone receptors [222]. Similarly, Youk et al [228], in a series of 166 invasive cancers, found that high elasticity values correlated with negative oestrogen and progesterone receptors (respectively, 162.1 ± 52 vs 139.6 ± 47.8,j9 = *0.015;* 162.5 ± 48.8 vs 136.6 ± 48.7,^ = *0.002).*

On the other hand, Ganau and Hayashi found no significant difference between elasticity values and hormone receptors [229, 230].

8.1.5. HER2 overexpression

HER2 overexpression is a poor prognostic factor, a predictive factor for response to anti-HER2 therapies, and a predictive factor for relative resistance to hormonal treatment (by crossover between oestrogen and HER2 receptor transduction pathways). This subtype of cancer benefits from 'targeted' therapies, treatments directed against relatively specific molecular anomalies in cancer cells, in this case molecules targeting the HER2 receptor family.

Some studies have looked at the correlation between elastography and HER2 receptor overexpression [223,230,231] and concluded that there was no significant difference between hardness and HER2 overexpression. We found similar results (all elastographic parameters $p > 0.05$).

8.1.6. Ki 67

The Ki-67 index is used to assess the rate of tumour cell proliferation, which is one of the most important prognostic parameters in breast cancer [1]. The Ki-67 index is determined immunohistochemically counting the percentage of cells positively labelled with the Ki-67 antigen, using the MIB-1 antibody [232].

The mean value of Ki-67 positive cells in breast tumours is 15%. This figure correlates with grade, reaching the highest values in poorly differentiated tumours [233].

Ki-67 is an essential marker for distinguishing between luminal A and B and consequently the type of treatment. Additional imaging information on Ki-67 status may be useful.

Liu et al. retrospectively studied the hardness of 82 luminal invasive cancers on elastography by correlating the Ki-67 status. They described a significant association between the mean elasticity ratio and a high Ki-67, greater than or equal to 14 (mean elasticity ratio of 5.83 for cancers with a high Ki-67 and 4.72 for

cancers with a low Ki-67₅ⱼp = *0.003*) [234].
In contrast, Ganau and Hayashi found no significant difference between elasticity values and Ki-67 [229, 230]. Our results are similar to theirs (all elastographic parameters $p > 0.05$).
Further studies with a larger sample size are required.

8.1.7. Molecular classification

Breast cancer is a heterogeneous disease with clinically relevant subgroups with their own prognostic impact [235].
Over the last decade, expression have made it possible to define tumours with different prognoses, paving the way for therapeutic strategies tailored to the tumour profile, and even predicting whether or not there will be a response to chemotherapy.
In imaging, in addition to characterising a mass and classifying it as an ACR BI-RADS category, it is becoming important to know the predictive features of an aggressive tumour subtype in order organise the fastest possible management for the patient.
In recent years, a number of studies have been carried out assess the relationship between tumour hardness measured by elastography and the molecular subtypes of invasive breast cancer [214, 217, 221, 222, 219, 229-234, 236-240]. These studies revealed divergent results.
In our study, triple-negative cancers were the hardest compared with the other molecular classes and luminal A subtype was the least hard compared with the other molecular subtypes ($p = 0.014$). Cancers with a high evolutionary potential (HER 2 and triple-negative) had a higher lesion hardness than cancers with a low evolutionary potential (luminal A and B).
Our results are in agreement with those reported Chang et al [222] who evaluated 377 patients with invasive breast cancer and their mean elasticity values. lis found that the elasticity values of triple-negative and HER2 tumours were higher than those of luminal subtypes A and B ($p < 0.0001$). lis showed that tumours with mean elasticity < 50 kPa were luminal subtypes.
In the Youk et al study [228], on a series of 166 invasive breast cancers in 152 patients, the authors also showed that invasive HER2 and triple-negative cancers were harder than luminal subtype cancers (mean elasticity of triple-negative tumours 163.1 ± 47.6 kPa vs luminal A 135.2 ±48.4kPa₅dp = *0.009*).
In the Evans et al. series, HER2 and triple-negative tumours had higher elasticity values (160.3 ± 56.2 kPa and 169.1 ± 48.5 kPa respectively) than luminal tumours (136.9 ± 57.2). According to Evans, tissue hardness appears to be statistically significantly correlated with tumour aggressiveness [217].
Furthermore, our results clearly differ from those reported by Ganau et al [229] who reported that aggressive phenotypes (triple-negative and HER2 status) seem to have a moderately lower elasticity than the least aggressive phenotypes (luminal A and luminal B), but without any significant difference.

Denis et al [231] reported that the triple-negative subtype had the lowest elasticity values (44.6 kPa triple-negative vs 108 kPa luminal A).
Similarly, Jin Y et al [214] found that the lowest elasticity ratio values were for triple-negative and HER2 tumours, 75.58 and 79.39 respectively. The highest values were for luminal subtypes A and B, 90.69 and 81.86 respectively ($p < 0.0001$). According to Jin, tumour hardness correlates with desmoplastic response, which is high in luminal subtype A.

8.1.8. Fibrosis vs. necrosis

In our study, tumour hardness correlated with the abundance of fibro-hyaline tumour stroma in malignant tumours (r - 0.5. y= *0.005*). This is in agreement with the in vivo study by Chamming's et al. who found a good correlation between tumour hardness and fibrosis rate (r = 0.83,y < *0.0001*) [241].
In contrast, Chamming's et al [241] negatively correlated hardness and tumour necrosis rate ($r = -0.76, p = 0.0004$). In contrast to our study, we found that elasticity ratio values were higher in necrotic lesions than in lesions without tumour necrosis.
The high hardness values of tumours with foci of necrosis in our series were explained by the fact that these tumours were of high grade and of the HER2 molecular subtype, which in our study had high elasticity ratio values. The number of necrotic tumours was too small to give a definitive conclusion. Further studies with a larger cohort are required.

8.1.9. Emboli

They are more often lymphatic than blood-related. They are found at the periphery of the tumour and are indicated by the abnormal presence of epithelial cells in the vascular lumens. When in doubt, the pathologist can use immunostaining. Lymphatic invasion is thought to be a predictive factor for local recurrence after conservative treatment and for distant relapse [242].
In our series, the hardness of invasive cancers correlated significantly with lymphatic invasion ($p = 0.04$).
Although little causality exists in our series, our current data may support the findings of Evans et al. who reported that tumour hardness was an independent predictor of the presence of vascular emboli [217].
Youk et al. reported that among the factors that influenced tumour hardness in shear wave elastography invasive cancers in 152 patients was lymphovascular invasion (187.9 kPa vs 138.3 kPa$_{5j}$p = *0.002*) [228].

8.1.10. Metastatic lymph nodes

According to basic research results, tumour hardness is increased in metastatic tumours [243].
Evans et al [217] reported that tumour hardness was an independent predictor of lymph node metastases in 396 invasive breast cancers.
Hayashi et al, reported that tumour hardness of invasive cancers on static

elastography correlated with metastatic axillary nodes in 503 patients with invasive breast cancer *($p < 0.0001$)* [230].

However, Youk et al., in a series of 166 invasive breast cancers in 152 patients, found no correlation between tumour hardness and metastatic involvement of axillary lymph nodes *($p = 0.662$)* [228]. A similar result was found in our study *($p = 0.23$).*

8.1. 11 Elastographic size versus histological size

We have shown that the elastographic size of malignant lesions was closer to the histological size, whereas ultrasound in B mode tended to underestimate it [244-247]. Approaching the true size pre-treatment represents a very important issue in the choice of treatment and could reduce the number of repeat surgeries for margins not in sano. To the best of our knowledge, there is no other publication correlating elastographic size and histological size.

Conclusion

Doctors have always associated certain diseases with variations in tissue consistency, particularly malignant tumours, which are described as being harder than the surrounding tissue. This empirical observation gave rise to the oldest diagnostic method, palpation. Technological developments gave rise to elastography.

The term elastography is used to describe a range of techniques that give relative information about tissue hardness. Ultrasound elastographic imaging techniques reproduce the same type of method as palpation, the tissues are compressed and their response to deformation is measured using ultrasound.

In this study, we were able to show that the hardness of a lesion constitutes a veritable indirect 'imprint' of the tumour. High lesion hardness appeared to be linked to tumour size ($p = 0.001$) and whether or not a lesion was mammographically visible ($p < 0.0001$).

We were able to demonstrate that significantly elevated values of elastographic parameters were in favour of malignancy ($p < 0.0001$).

We also found that hardness was significantly higher in infiltrating cancers than in in situ cancers ($p < 0.0001$), *in* high-grade cancers rather than low-grade ($p = 0.017$) and in tumours with high evolutionary potential than in tumours with low evolutionary potential φ- *0.014).* On the other hand, we showed that the elastographic size was closer to the histological size (27.26 mm vs 27.03 mm, respectively) than to the size measured in B-mode ultrasound (23.21 mm).

In our study, although the sensitivity of ultrasound is high (100%), the specificity of elastography is significantly higher (97.65%) than that of B-mode ultrasound (25.5%). These results imply that elastography is a simple, non-invasive and rapid diagnostic method that can make a diagnostic contribution to B-mode ultrasound by increasing specificity, thereby reducing the false-positive rate. It can also help to reclassify BIRADS 3 lesions as BIRADS 2, in order reduce the number of unnecessary follow-ups (98.01%), but also to reduce the rate of unnecessary biopsies (79.28%), patient anxiety and finally to help reduce the cost of biopsy.

Thus, it can be argued that the addition of elastography to B mode ultrasound could help the radiologist to refine his diagnostic criteria and his interpretation of breast lesions.

Recommendations

Breast elastography is a valuable complementary ultrasound technique for characterising breast masses. It improves the specificity of B-mode imaging, thereby reducing the need for close follow-up and sampling of benign lesions.
This technique has the advantage of rapidity (use the same ultrasound probe, examination time of a few minutes) and safety, which should make it a routine examination integrated into the diagnostic decision algorithm (fig. 84). Allowing more specific management of certain breast lesions.

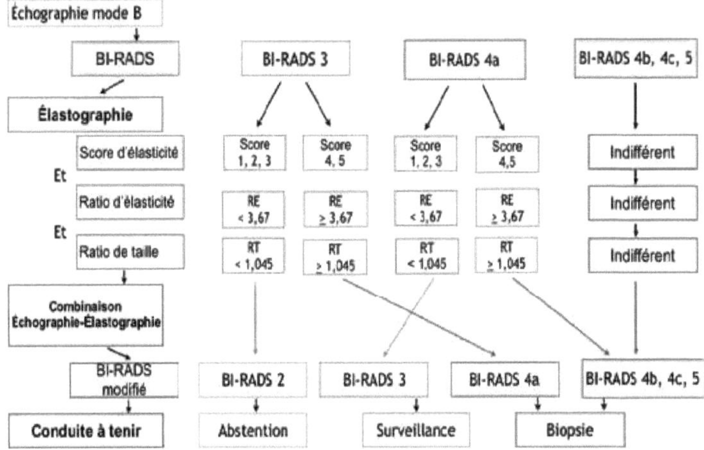

Fig. 84. Diagnostic decision algorithm for breast masses.

References

1. Levy L, Michelin J, Teman G, Martin B, Dana A, Lacan A, Meyer D. Techniques d'exploration radiologique du sein (mammographie, échographie, IRM). Encycl Méd Chir 2001; 34-800-A-10.
2. Banks, E., Reeves, G., Beral, V., Bull, D., Crossley, B., Simmonds, M., . . Patnick, J. Influence of personal characteristics of individual women on sensitivity and specificity of mammography in the Million Women Study: Cohort study. BMJ, 2004; 329, 477-482.
3. Heywang-Kobrunner S H, Schreer I, Bassler R, Perlet C, Viehweg P. Mammography. Imagerie diagnostique du sein : Mammographie, échographie, IRM, techniques interventionnelles 2007 ; 19-97.
4. Barry DA, Cronin KA, Plevritis SK, Fryback DG,Clarke L, Zelen M, et al. Effect of screening and adjuvant therapy on mortality from breast cancer. N Emgl J Med. 2005;353 (17): 1784-92.
5. Tabar L, Yen MF, Vitak B, Chen H-HT, Smith RA, Duffy SW. Mammography service screening and martality in breast cancer patients: 20-year follow-up before and after introduction of screening. 1ANCET. 2003; 361 (9367) : 1405-10.
6. Hellquist BN, Duffy SW, Abdsaleh S, Bjomeld L, Bordas P, Tabar L, et al. Effectiveness of population-based service screening with mammography forwomen ages 40 to 49 years evaluation of the Swedish Mammography in Y oung Women (SCRY) cohort. Cancer. 2011 ; 117 (4): 714-22.
7. Kerlikowske K, Grady D, Barclay J, Sickles EA, Ernster V. Effect of age, breast density, and Family history on the sensitivity of first screening mammography. JAMA. 1996; 276 (1) : 33-8.
8. Mandelson M, oestreicher N, Porter PL,White D, Finder CA, Taplin SH, et al. Breast density as a predictor of mammographic detection: comparison of interval and screen detected cancers. J Natl Cancer Inst. 2000; 92 (13): 1081-7.
9. Leconte I, Feger C, Galant C, Berlére M, Berg BV, D'Hoore W, et aal. Mammography and subsequent whole breast sonography of non palpable breast cancers: the importance of radiologie breast density. AJR AmJ Roentgenol. 2003; 180 (6) : 1675-9.
10. D'Orsi CJ et al. ACR BI-RADS ® Atlas, Breast Imaging Reporting and Data System. Reston, VA, American College of Radiology; 2013.
11. Chee, Y. L., Crawford, J. C., Watson, H. G., & Greaves, M. (2008). Guidelines on the assessment of bleeding risk prior to surgery or invasive procedures. British Journal of Haematology, 140(5), 496-504.
12. Stavros AT, Thickman D, Rapp CL, Dennis MA, Parker SH, Sisney GA. Solid breast nodules: use of sonography to distinguish between benign and malignant lesions. Radiology. 1995 Jul; 196 (l):123-34.
13. Mitka, M. (). New ultrasound elasticity technique may reduce need for breast biopsies. The Journal of the American Medical Association. 2007; 297(5), 453-458.
14. Zonderland HM,Pope TL,Nieborg AJ. The positive predictive value of the breast imaging reporting and data system (BI-RADS) as a method of Quality assessment in breast imaging in a hospital populatio. Eur Radiol. 2004; 14 (10) : 1743-50.
15. Orel SG, Kay N, Reynolrs C, Sullivan DC. BI-RADS categorization as s predictor of malignancy. Radiology . 1999; 211 (3): 845-50.
16. Liberman L, Abramson AF, Squires FB, Glassman JR, Morris EA, Dershaw DD. The breast imaging reporting and data system: positive predictive value of mammographic features and final assessment categories. AJR Am J Roentgenol. 1998; 171 (1) : 35-40.
17. Kim EK, Ko KH, Oh KK, Kwak JY, Kim MJ, et al. Clinical application of the BI-RADS final assessment to breast sonography in conjunction with mammography. AJR AmJ Roentgenol. 2008; 190 (5) : 1209-15.
18. Hamy AS, Giacchetti S, Albiter M, de Bazelaire C, Cuvier C, Perret F, et al BI-RADS

categorisation of 2,708 consecutive nonpalpable breast lesions in patients referred to a dedicated breast care unit. Eur Radiol. 2012; 22 (1): 9-17.

19. Lamb PM, Perry NM, Vinnicombe SJ, Wells CA. Correlation between ultrasound characteristics, mammographic findings and histological grade in patients with invasive ductal carcinoma of the breast. Clin Radiol. 2000; 55 (1): 40-4.

20. Boné B, Aspelin P, Bronge L, Isberg B, Perbeck L, Veress B. Sensitivity and specificity of MRmammography with histopathological correlation in 250 breasts. Acta Radiol Stockh Swed 1987. 1996; 37 (2) : 208-13.

21. Stamper PC, Herman S, Klippenstein DL, Winston JS, Edge SB, Arredondo MA, et al. Suspect breast lesions: findings at dymamic gadolonium-enhaced MR imaging correlated with mammographic and pathologic features. Radiology. 1995 : 197 (2) : 387-95.

22. Sung H, Ferlay J, Siegel RL et al. Global cancer statistics 2020: GLOBOCAN estimates of incidence and mortality worldwide for 36 cancers in 185 countries. *CA Cancer J Clin.* 2021;71:209-249.

23. K. Bouzid, Breast cancer. Le fascicule de la sauté, 2004, 2011

24. Ministry of Health and Population, National Institute of Public Health. Registre des tumeurs d' Alger, année 2015 (www.sante.dz/insp/registre-tumeurs-alger-2015.pdf).

25. M Hamdi Cherif, A Mahnane, S Laouamri, Z. Zaidi et all. Cancer registry of Sétif (Algeria): incidence, trend and survival 1986-2010.

26. L Mokhtari, N Midoun et al. Oran Cancer Registry, 13th report, March 2006 (1996-2006).

27. K.Meguenni.al. Tlemcen cancer registry. Tlemcen: l'unité d'information sanitaire et biostatistiques du CHU Tedjini Damerdji de Tlemcen, 2012. 37

28. Abid L. Cancer epidemiology in Algeria: best use of cancer registers. J Afr Cancer 2009;1:98-103.

29. Hamdi Cherif M, Guerra D, Abdellouche D et al. Cancer incidence in Sétif 1998- 2002. In: Curado MP, Edwards B, Shin HR, Storm H, Ferlay J, Heanue M, Boyle P eds. Cancer incidence in five continents, vol.IX. Lyon, IARC Scientific Publications No 160, 2008.

30. Barra FR, Ribeiro AC, Mathieu DO, Rodrigues AC. Angiomammography: examination protocol. Journal of Diagnostic and Interventional Radiology 2014; 95, 351-352.

31. American College of Radiology (ACR). Illustrated Breast Imaging reporting and data system (BIRADS TM). 2nd ed Reston, VA; 1998.

32. Balleyguiera C, Thomassin-Naggarac I. BI-RADS 2013 in mammography: a short guide to what's new. Imagerie de la Femme, 2015; 25, 1-7

33. Corsetti V, Houssami N, Ferrari A, Ghirardi M, Bellarosa S, Angelini O, et al. Breast screening with ultrasound in women with mammography-negative dense breasts: evidence on incremental cancer detection and false positives, and associated cost. Eur J Cancer. 2008 Mar;44(4):539-44.

34. Athanasiou A, Tardivon A, Ollivier L, Thibault F, El Khoury C, Neuenschwander S. How to optimize breast ultrasound. Eur J Radiol. 2009 Jan;69(l):6-13.

35. Weinstein SP, Conant EF, Sehgal C. Technical advances in breast ultrasound imaging. Semin Ultrasound CT MR. 2006 Aug;27(4):273-83.

36. Sehgal CM, Weinstein SP, Arger PH, Conant EF. A review of breast ultrasound. J Mammary Gland Biol Neoplasia. 2006 Apr; 11 (2): 113-23.

37. Amersham Health. Encyclopaedia of Medical Imaging. http://eu.aershamhealth/com/medcyclopaedia/

38. Clevert DA, Jung EM, Jungius KP, Ertan K, Kubale R. Value of tissue harmonic imaging (THI) and contrast harmonic imaging (CHI) in detection and characterisation of breast tumours. Eur Radiol 2007 ; 17 : 1-10.

39. Rosen EL, Soo MS. Tissue harmonic imaging sonography of breast lesions: improved margin analysis, conspicuity, and image quality compared to conventional ultrasound. Clin Imaging. 2001

Nov-Dec;25(6):379-84.
40. Athanasiou A, Balleyguier C. New techniques in breast ultrasound. Imagerie de la Femme. 2007;17(4):247-54.
41. Huber S, Wagner M, Medi M, Czembirek H. Real-time spatial compound imaging in breast ultrasound. Ultrasound Med Biol 2002; 28: 155-63.
42. Cha JH, Moon WK, Cho N, Chung SY, Park SH, Park JM, et al. Differentiation of benign from malignant solid breast masses: conventional US versus compound imaging. Radiology 2005;237:841-6.
43. Balu-Maestro C. Bases de l'échographie mammarie. Imager ie du sein. Paris : Elsevier-Masson ; 2012. p. 101-17.
44. Cosgrove DO, Keddar RP, Bamber JC, Al-Murrani B, Davey JB, Fischer C, et al. Color US in differential diagnosis. Radiology 1993; 189(l):99-104.
45. Raza S, Baum JK. Solid breast lesions: evaluation with power Doppler US. Radiology 1997; 2O3'l):164 -8.
46. Lee SW, Choi HY, Baek SY, Lim SM. Role of color and power doppler imaging in differentiating between malignant and benign solid breast masses. J Clin Ultrasound. 2002 Oct; 30 (8):459-64.
47. Daly CP, Bailey JE, Klein KA, Helvie MA. Complicated breast cysts on sonography: is aspiration necessary to exclude malignancy? Acad Radiol. 2008 May;15(5):610-7.
48. Hong AS, Rosen EL, Soo MS, Baker JA. BI-RADS for sonography: positive and negative predictive values of sonographic features. AJR Am J Roentgenol. 2005 Apr; 184(4): 12605.
49. Graf O, Helbich TH, Fuchsjaeger MH, et al. Follow-up of palpable circumscribed noncalcified solid breast masses at mammography and US: can biopsy be averted? Radiology 2004; 233(3):850-856.
50. Berg WA, Sechtin AG, Marques H, Zhang Z. Cyctic breast masses and the ACRIN 6666 experience. Radiol Clin North Am 2010; 48(5): 931-87.
51. Mainiero MB, Goldkamp A, Lazarus E, et al. Characterization of breast masses with sonography: can biopsy of some solid masses be deferred? J Ultrasound Med 2005;24(2):161-167.
52. Lazarus E, Mainiero MB, Schepps B, Koelliker SL, Livingston LS. BI-RADS lexicon for US and mammography: interobserver variability and positive predictive value. Radiology. 2006 May;239(2):385-91.
53. Raza S, Goldkamp AL, Chikarmane SA, Birdwell RL. US of breast masses categorized as BIRADS 3, 4 and 5: pictorial review of factors influencing clinical management. Radiographics 2010; 30 (5): 1199-213.
54. Brigitte M, Kamina P; Surgical anatomy of the breast Breast cancer. Elsevier Masson; 2007; 2-10.
55. Lee HJ, Kim EK, Kim MJ, Y ouk JH, Lee JY, Kang DR, et al. Observer variability of Breast Imaging Reporting and Data System (BI-RADS) for breast ultrasound. Eur J Radiol. 2008 Feb;65(2):293-8.
56. Park CS, Lee JH, Yim HW, Kang BJ, Kim HS, Jung JI, et al. Observer agreement using the ACR Breast Imaging Reporting and Data System (BI-RADS)- ultrasound, First Edition (2003). Korean J Radiol. 2007 Sep-Oct;8(5):397-402.
57. Berg WA, Blume JD, Cormack JB, Mendelson EB. Operator dependence ofphysician-performed whole-breast US: lesion detection and characterization. Radiology. 2006 Nov;241(2):355-65.
58. Skaane P. Ultrasonography as adjunct to mammography in the evaluation of breast tumors. Acta Radiol Suppl. 1999;420:1-47.
59. Dickinson RJ, Hill CR. Measurement of soft tissue motion using correlation between A-scans.Ultrasound Med Biol 1982;8(3):263-71.

60. Krouskop TA, Dougherty DR, Vinson FS. A pulsed Doppler ultrasonic system for making noninvasive measurements of the mechanical properties of soft tissue. J Rehabil Res Dev 1987;24(2):l-8.
61. Ophir J, Céspedes I, Ponnekanti H, Yazdi Y, Li X. Elastography: a quantitative method for imaging the elasticity of biological tissues. Ultrason Imaging 1991;13(2):lll-34.
62. Eisenscher A et al. Rhythmic echographic palpation. Echosismography. A new technique of differentiating benign and malignant tumors by ultrasonic study of tissue elasticity. J Radiol 1983;64(4):255-61.
63. Cespedes I et al. Elastography: elasticity imaging using ultrasound with application to muscle and breast in vivo. Ultrason Imaging 1993;15(2):73-88.
64. Booi RC, Carson PL, O'Donnell M, Roubidoux MA, Hall AL, Rubin JM. Characterization of cysts using differential correlation coefficient values from two dimensional breast elastography: preliminary study. Ultrasound Med Biol. 2008 Jan;34 (1): 12-21.
65. Leong LC, Sim LS, Lee YS, Ng FC, Wan CM, Fook-Chong SM, et al. A prospective study to compare the diagnostic performance of breast elastography versus conventional breast ultrasound. Clin Radiol. 2010 Nov;65(ll):887-94.
66. Moon WK, Chang SC, Huang CS, Chang RF. Breast tumor classification using fuzzy clustering for breast elastography. Ultrasound Med Biol. 2011 May;37(5):700-8.
67. Garra BS. Elastography: current status, future prospects, and making it work for you. Ultrasound Q. 2011 Sep;27(3): 177-86.
68. Sewell CW. Pathology of benign and malignant breast disorders. Radiol Clin North Am 1995; 33 (6): 1067-80.
69. Sarvazyan A, Skovoroda AR, Emelianov S, Fowlkes JB, Biophysical bases of elasticity imaging. Acoust Imaging 1995; 21: 223-41.
70. Goddi A, Bonardi M, Alessi S, et al. Breast elastography: a literature review. Journal of Ultrasound 2012; 15:192-8.
71. Royer D and Dieulesaint E, Elastic Waves in Solids I: Free and Guided Propagation. 2000.
72. Gennison JL, Deffieux T, Fink M, Tanter M. Ultrasonic elastography: principles and procedures. Journal of Diagnostic and Interventional Radiology ,2013 ,94, 504-513.
73. Krouskop TA, Wheeler TM, Kallel F, Garra BS, Hall T. Elastic moduli of breast and prostate tissues under compression. Ultrason Imaging. 1998 Oct;20(4):260-74.
74. Khaled W, Reichling S, Bruhns OT, Ermert H. Ultrasonic strain imaging and reconstructive elastography for biological tissue. Ultrasonics. 2006 Dec 22;44 Suppl l:el99-202.
75. Sinkus R, Bercoff J, Tanter M, Gennisson JL, El-Khoury C, Servois V, et al. Nonlinear viscoelastic properties of tissue assessed by ultrasound. IEEE Trans Ultrason Ferroelectr Freq Control. 2006 Nov;53(U):2009-18.
76. Nightingale K, Soo MS, Nightingale R, Trahey G. Acoustic radiation force impulse imaging: in vivo demonstration of clinical feasibility. Ultrasound Med Biol. 2002 Feb;28(2):227-35, version 1-22 May 2013.
77. Dietrich FC, Barr RG, Farrokh A, Dighe M, Hocкe M, et al. Strain Elastography - How To Do It?". Ultrasound Int Open 2017; 3: E 137-E 149.
78. Sigrist R, Liau J, El Kaffas A, Chammas MC, Willmann JK. Ultrasound Elastography: Review of Techniques and Clinical Applications. Theranostics 2017, Vol. 7, Issue 5.
79. Barr RG. The Role of Sonoelastography in Breast Lesions. Semin Ultrasound CT MRI 39:98-105 C 2018 Elsevier.
80. Guo R, Lu G, Qin B, Fei B. Ultrasound imaging technologies for breast cancer detection and management: A review. Ultrasound in Med. & Biol, Vol. 44, No. 1, pp. 37-70, 2018.
81. Xiao Y, Zeng J, Zhang X, Niu L, Qian M, Wang, CZ, et al. UltrasoundStrain Elastography for Breast Lesions. J Ultrasound Med 2017; 36:1089-1100.
82. Bercoff J, Chaffai S, Tanter M, Sandrin L, Catheline S, Fink M, et al. In vivo breast tumor

detection using transient elastography. Ultrasound Med Biol. 2003 Oct;29(10): 1387-96.
83. Garra BS, Cespedes El, Ophir J, Spratt SR, Zuurbier RA, Magnant CM, et al. Elastography of breast lesions: initial clinical results. Radiology. 1997 Jan;202(l):79-86.
84. Itoh A, Ueno E, Tohno E, Kamma H, Takahashi H, Shiina T, et al. Breast disease: clinical application of US elastography for diagnosis. Radiology. 2006 May;239(2):341-50.
85. Farrokh A, Wojcinski S, Degenhardt F, et al. Diagnostic value of strain ratio measurement in the differentiation of malignant and benign breast lesions. Ultraschall in der Medizin 2011;32:400-5.
86. Thomas A, Degenhardt F, Farrokh A, et al. Significant differentiation of focal breast lesions: calculation of strain ratio in breast sonoelastography. Academic Radiology 2010;17(5):558-63.
87. Zhi H, Xiao XY,Yang HY, Ou B, Wen YL, Luo BM. Ultrasonic elastography in breast cancer diagnosis: strain ratio vs 5-point scale. Acad Radiol. 2010 Oct;17(10):1227-33.
88. Ginat DT, Destounis SV, Barr RG, Castaneda B, Strang JG, Rubens DJ. US elastography of breast and prostate lesions. Radiographics. 2009 Nov;29(7):2007-16.
89. Barr RG. Real-time ultrasound elasticity of the breast: initial clinical results. Ultrasound Quarterly 2010; 26(2):61-6.
90. Regner DM, Hesley GK, Hangiandreou NJ, et al. Breast lesions: evaluation with US strain imaging-clinical experience of multiple observers. Radiology 2006;238:425-37.
91. Landoni V, Francione V, Marzi S, et al. Quantitative analysis of elastography images in the detection of breast cancer. European Journal of Radiology 2011 ;81 (7): 1527-31.
92. Tardivon A, El Khoury C, Thibault F, Wyler A, Barreau B, Neuenschwander S. Elastography of the breast: a prospective study of 122 lesions. J Radiol 2007;88:657-62.
93. Zhi H, Ou B, Luo BM, Feng X, Wen YL, Yang HY. Comparison of ultrasound elastography, mammography, and sonography in the diagnosis of solid breast lesions. J Ultrasound Med 2007;26(6):807-15.
94. Moon WK, Huang CS, Shen WC, Takada E, Chang RF, Joe J, et al. Analysis of elastographic and B-mode features at sonoelastography for breast tumor classification. Ultrasound Med Biol 2009;35(ll): 1794-802.
95. Tardivon A, Delignette A, Lemery S, Baratte B, Levy L, David P, et al. Ultrasound elastography: results of a French multicentric prospective study about 345 breast lesions. Oral communication ECR Vienna 2-6 March 2006. Euro J Radiol, Abstract B-344.
96. Cho N, Moon WK, Kim HY, Chang JM, Park SH, Lyou CY. Sonoelastographic strain index for differentiation of benign and malignant non palpable breast masses. J Ultrasound Med. 2010 Jan;29(l): 1-7.
97. Scaperrotta G, Ferranti C, Costa C, Mariani L, Marchesini M, Suman L, et al. Role of sonoelastography in non-palpable breast lesions. Eur Radiol 2008;18(ll):2381-9.
98. Thomas A, Fischer T, Frey H, Ohlinger R, Grunwald S, Blohmer JU, et al. A Real-time elastography-an advanced method of ultrasound: first results in 108 patients with breast lesions. Ultrasound Obstet Gynecol 2006;28:335-40.
99. Bercoff J, Chaffai S, Tanter M, et al. In vivo breast tumors detection using transient elastography. Ultrasound in Medicine and Biology 2003;29: 1387-96.
100. Bercoff J., "L'imagerie échographique ultrarapide et son application à l'étude de la viscoélasticité du corps humain," Université Paris VII Denis Diderot, 2004.
101 Gennisson JL, Renier M, Catheline S, Barriere C, Bercoff J, Tanter M, et al. Acoustoelasticity in soft solids: assessment of the nonlinear shear modulus with the acoustic radiation force. J Acoust Soc Am. 2007 Dec;122(6):3211-9.
102 Athanasiou A, Tardivon A, Tanter M, Sigal-Zafrani B, Bercoff J, Deffieux T, et al. Breast lesions: quantitative elastography with supersonic shear imaging-preliminary results. Radiology. 2010 Jul;256(l):297-303.
103 Baileyguier C, Canale S, Ben Hassen W, et al. Breast elasticity: principles, technique, results:

an update and overview of commercially available software. European Journal of Radiology 2012.
104 .Tanter M, Bercoff J, Athanasiou A, Deffieux T, Gennisson JL, Montaldo G, et al. Quantitative assessment of breast lesion viscoelasticity: initial clinical results using supersonic shear imaging. Ultrasound Med Biol. 2008 Sep;34(9): 1373-86.
105 .Bercoff J, Tanter M, Fink M. Supersonic shear imaging: a new technique for soft tissue elasticity mapping. IEEE Trans Ultrason Ferroelectr Freq Control 2004; 51:396-409.
106 Evans A, Whelehan P, Thomson K, et al. Differentiating benign from malignant solid breast masses: value of shear wave elastography according to lesion stiffness combined with grey scale ultrasound according to BI-RADS classification. British Journal of Cancer 2012;107:224-9
107 Balu-Maestro C, Chapellier C, Ettore F, Juhan V, Athanasiou A, Tardivon A, et al. Shear wave elastography of breast lesions Imagerie de la Femme, Volume 21, Issue 3, September 2011, Pages 105-110.
108 Nightingale K, Bentley R, Trahey G. Observations of tissue response to acoustic radiation force: opportunities for imaging. Ultrason Imaging. 2002 Jul;24(3): 129-38.
109 Nightingale KR, Paimeri ML, Nightingale RW, Trahey GE. On the feasibility of remote palpation using acoustic radiation force. J Acoust Soc Am. 2001 Jul;110(l):625-34.
110 Nightingale KR, Nightingale RW, Paimeri ML, Trahey GE. A finite element model of remote palpation of breast lesions using radiation force: factors affecting tissue displacement. Ultrason Imaging. 2000 Jan;22(l):35-54.
111 Li PC, Lee WN. An efficient speckle tracking algorithm for ultrasonic imaging.Ultrason Imaging. 2002 Oct;24(4):215-28.version 1-22 May 2013
112 . Jiang J, Hall TJ. A parallelizable real-time motion tracking algorithm with applications to ultrasonic strain imaging. Phys Med Biol. 2007 Jul 7;52 (13):3773-90.
113 Paimeri ML, Frinkley KD, Nightingale KR. Experimental studies of the thermal effects associated with radiation force imaging of soft tissue. Ultrason Imaging. 2004 Apr;26 (2):100-14.
114 Zhai L et al. An integrated indenter-ARFI imaging system for tissue stiffness quantification. Ultrason Imaging 2008;30(2):95-lll.
115 Nightingale K, McAleavey S, Trahey G. "Shear-wave generation using acoustic radiation force: in vivo and ex vivo results". Ultrasound in Medicine & Biology, vol. 29, no. 12, pp. 1715-23,2003.
116 Tozaki M, Isobe S, Fukuma E. Preliminary study of ultrasonographic tissue quantification of the breast using the acoustic radiation force impulse (ARFI) technology. Eur J Radiol. 2011 Nov;80(2):el82-7.
117 .Tozaki M, Isobe S, Sakamoto M, et al. Combination of elastography and tissue quantification using the acoustic radiation force impulse (ARFI) technology for differential diagnosis ofbreast masses. Japanese Journal of Radiology 2012;30(8):659-70.
118 Meng W, Zhang G, Wu C, Wu G, Song Y, Lu Z. Preliminary results of acoustic radiation force impulse (ARFI) ultrasound imaging ofbreast lesions. Ultrasound Med Biol. 2011 Sep;37(9): 1436-43.
119 .Bai M, Du L, Gu J, et al. Virtual touch tissue quantification using acoustic radiation force impulse technology: initial clinical experience with solid breast masses. Journal of Ultrasound in Medicine 2012;31:289-94.
120 Balleyguier C., Ciolovan L., Ammari S., Canale S., Sethom S., Al Rouhbane R., Vielh P., Dromain C. Breast elastography: The technical process and its applications Diagnostic and Interventional Imaging, Volume 94, Issue 5, May 2013, P 519-530.
121 Zhu QL, Jiang YX, Liu JB, Liu H, Sun Q, Dai Q, et al. Real-time ultrasound elastography : its potential role in assessment of breast lesions. Ultrasound Med Biol 2008; 34(8): 12328.
122 Cespedes I et al. Elastography: elasticity imaging using ultrasound with application to muscle and breast in vivo. Ultrason Imaging 1993;15(2):73-88.
123 Sadigh G, Carlos RC, Neal CH, et al. Accuracy of quantitative ultrasound elastography for

differentiation of malignant and benign breast abnormalities: a meta-analysis. Breast Cancer Research and Treatment 2012; 134: 923- 31.
124 Bartow SA, Pathak DR, Black WC, et al. Prevalence of benign, atypical, and malignant breast lesions in populations at different risk for breast cancer. A forensic autopsy study. Cancer 1987;60:2751-60.
125 Garra BS. Imaging and estimation of tissue elasticity by ultrasound. Ultrasound Quarterly 2007;23(4):255- 68.
126 Raza S, Odulate A, Ong EM, et al. Using real-time tissue elastography for breast lesion evaluation: our initial experience. Journal of Ultrasound in Medicine 2010;29(4):551- 63.
127 Sewell CW. Pathology of benign and malignant breast disorders. Radiol Clin North Am 1995; 33 (6): 1067-80.
128.Tozaki M, Fukuma E. Pattem classification of shear wave elastography images for differential diagnosis between benign and malignant solid breast masses. Acta Radiologica 2011;52:1069- 75.
129.Tozaki M, Isobe S, Yamaguchi M, et al. Ultrasonographic elastography of the breast using acoustic radiation force impulse technology: preliminary study. Japanese Journal of Radiology 2011; 29(6):452- 6.
130.Berg WA, Cosgrove DO, Doré CJ, et al. Shear-wave elastography improves the specificity of breast US: The BEI multinational study of 939 masses. Radiology 2012;262(2):435- 49.
131 .Sohn YM, Kim MJ, Kim EK, et al. Sonographic elastography combined with conventional sonography how much is it helpful for diagnostic performance? .Journal of Ultrasound in Medicine 2009;28(4):413- 20.
132 Barr RG. Sonographic breast elastography: a primer. Journal of Ultrasound in Medicine 2012;31(5):773- 83.
133.Schaefer FKW, Heer I, Schaefer PJ, et al. Breast ultrasound elastography - results of 193 breast lesions in a prospective study with histopathologic correlation. European Journal of Radiology 20U;77(3):450- 6.
134 Regini E, Bagnerà S, Tota D, et al. Role of sonoelastography in characterizing breast nodules. Preliminary experience with 120 lesions. La Radiologia Medica 2010; 115:551- 62.
135.Stachs A, Hartmann S, Stubert J, et al. Differentiating between malignant and benign breast masses: factors limiting sonoelastographic strain ratio. Ultra-schall Med. 2013, 34 (2): 131-136.
136 .Popiel M, Mróz-Klimas D, Kasprzak R, et al. Mammary carcinoma - current diagnostic methods and symptomatology in imaging studies. Polish Journal of Radiology 2012;77(4):35- 44.
137 .Hayashi M, Yamamoto Y, Ibusuki M, et al. Evaluation of tumor stiffness by elastography is predictive for pathologic complete response to neoadjuvant chemotherapy in patients with breast cancer. Annals of Surgical Oncology 2012;19(9):3042- 9.
138 Mori M, Tsunoda H, Kawauchi N, et al. Elastographic evaluation of mucinous carcinoma of the breast. Breast Cancer 2012; 19 (l):60- 3.
139 Giuseppetti G, Martegani A, Di Cioccio B, Baldassarre S. Elastosonography in the diagnosis of the nodular breast lesions: preliminary report. La Radiologia Medica 2005;110:69- 76.
140 Lee JH, Kim SH, Kang BJ, et al. Role and clinical usefulness of elastography in small breast masses. Academic Radiology 2011;18:74- 80.
141 Yerli H, Yilmaz T, Kaskati T, et al. Qualitative and semiquantitative evaluations of solid breast lesions by sonoelastography. Journal of Ultrasound in Medicine 2011;30:179- 86.
142 Barr RG, Destounis S, Lackey 2nd LB, et al. Evaluation of breast lesions using sonographic elasticity imaging. A multicenter trial. Journal of Ultrasound in Medicine 2012;31(2):281- 7.
143 . Yoon JH, Kim MJ, Kim EK, Moon HJ, Choi JS. Discordant elastography images of breast lesions: how various factors lead to discoddant findings. Ultraschall Med 2012, http://dx.doi.org/10.1055/s- 0032-1312948.
144 Zhao QL, Ruan LT, Zhang H, et al. Diagnosis of solid breast lesions by elastography 5- point score and strain ratio method. European Journal of Radiology 2012;81(ll):3245- 9.

145 Varghese T, Konofagou EE, Ophir J, et al. Direct strain estimation in elastography using spectral cross-correlation. Ultrasound in Medicine and Biology 2000;26:1525- 37.
146 Ciurea AI, Bolboac SD, Ciortea CA, et al. The influence of technical factors on sonoelastographic assessment of solid breast nodules. Ultraschall in der Medizin 2011;32:S27-34
147 Chang JM, Moon WK, Cho N, et al. Breast mass evaluation: factors influencing the quality of US elastography. Radiology 2011;259:59- 64.\
148 Berg WA, Blume JD, Cormack JB, Mendelson EB, Lehrer D, Bohm-Velez M, et al. Combined screening with ultrasound and mammography vs mammography alone in women at elevated risk of breast cancer. JAMA. 2008 May 14;299(18):2151-63
149 Ancelle-Park R, Paty AC, Julien M et al. Les cancers détectés par le nouveau cahier des charges et leur classification selon le code BI-RADS de L'ACR 27 ernes joumées de la Société française de sénologie et de pathologie mammaire. Deauville 16-18 November 2005. www.senologie.com .
150 Lazarus E, Mainiero MB, Schepps B, Koelliker SL, Livingston LS. BI-RADS lexicon for US and mammography: interobserver variability and positive predictive value. Radiology. 2006 May;239(2):385-91.
151 Jacobs TW, Chen YY, Guinee Jr DG, Holden JA, Chai, Bauermeister DE, et al. Fibroepithelial lesions with cellular stroma on breast core needle biopsy: are therepredictors of outcome on surgical excision? Am J Clin Pathol 2005;124:342-54.
152 Youden WJ. Index for rating diagnostic tests. Cancer. 1950; 3: 32±35. PMID: 15405679
153 Gong X, Xu Q, Xu Z, et al. Real-time elastography for the differentiation of benign and malignant breast lesions: a meta-analysis. Breast Cancer Research and Treatment 2011;130(l):ll-8.
154 Stoian D, Timar B, Craina M, Bemad E, Petrel, Craciunescu M. Qualitative strain elastography - strain ratio evaluation - an important tool in breast cancer diagnosis. Med Ultrason 2016, Vol. 18, no. 2, 195-200.
155 Khamis M, Alaa El-deen AM, Abdel Azim Ismail A. The diagnostic value of sonoelastographic strain ratio in discriminating malignant from benign solid breast masses. The Egyptian Journal of Radiology and Nuclear Medicine 48 (2017) 1149-1157.
156 .Navarro B, Ubeda B, Vallespi M, Wolf C et al (2011) Role of elastography in the assessment of breast lesions: preliminary results. J Ultrasound Med 30:313-321.
157 Menezes R, Sardessai S, Furtado R, Sardessai M. Correlation of Strain Elastography with Conventional Sonography and FNAC/Biopsy. Journal of Clinical and Diagnostic Research. 2016 Jul, Vol-10(7): TC05-TC10.
158 Arslan S, Uslu N, Ozturk FU, Akcay EY, Tezcaner T, Agildere AM. Can strain elastography combined with ultrasound breast imaging reporting and data system be a more effective method in the differentiation of benign and malignant breast lesions? J Med Ultrasonics 2017. DOI 10.1007/sl0396-017-0772-y.
159 Bojanic K, Katavic N, Smolic M, Peric M, Kralik K, Sikora M et al. Implementation of elastography score and strain ratio in combination with B-mode ultrasound avoids unnecessary biopsies of breast lesions. Ultrasound in Med. & Biol, Vol. 43, No. 4, pp. 804-816, 2017.
160 Houelleu Demay ML, Monghal C, Bertrand P, Vilde A, Brunereau L. An assessment of the performance of elastography for the investigation of BI-RADS 4 and BI-RADS 5 breast lesions: correlations with pathological anatomy findings. Diagn Interv Imaging 2012;93(10):757-66.
161 .Parajuly SS, Lan PY, Yun MB, Gang YZ, et al. Diagnostic potential of strain ratio measurement and a 5 point scoring method for detection of breast cancer: Chinese experience. Asian Pac J Cancer Prev 2012;13:1447-52.
162 Fischer T, Peisker U, Fiedor S, et al. Significant differentiation of focal breast lesions: raw data-based calculation of strain ratio. Ultraschall Med 2012;33:372-9.
163 Barr RG, Nakashima K, Amy D, et al. WFUMB guidelines and recommendations for clinical use of ultrasound elastography: Part 2: breast. Ultrasound Med Biol 2015;41(5):1148-1160

164 Jung NY, Park CS, Kim SH, Jung HS, et al. Sonoelastographic strain ratio: how does the position of reference fat influence it? Jpn J Radiol 2016;34 (6):440-7.
165 .Zhou J, Zhan W, Chang C et al (2013) Role of acoustic shear wave velocity measurement in characterization of breast lesions. Ultrasound Med 32:285-294.
166 Zhou J, Zhou C, Zhan W, Jia X, Dong Y, Yang Z. Elastography ultrasound for breast lesions: fat-to-lesion strain ratio vs glandto- lesion strain ratio. Eur Radiol 2014;24(12):3171-3177.5.
167 .Graziano L, Bitencourt A, Cohen M, Guatelli C et al Elastographic Evaluation of Indeterminate Breast Masses on Ultrasound. Thieme-Revinter, 2017. DOI http://dx.doi.org/ 10.1055/s-0036-1597753.
168 Redling K, Schwab F, Siebert M, Schötzau A, Zanetti-Dällenbach R. Elastography Complements Ultrasound as Principle Modality in Breast Lesion Assessment. Gynecol Obstet Invest 2016. DOI: 10.1159/000445746.
169 Balçik A, Polat AV, Bayrak ÌK, Polat AK. Efficacy of sonoelastography in distinguishing benign from malignant breast masses. J Breast Health 2016;12:37-43.
170 Dawooda MAA, Ibrahima N, Elsaeeda H, Hegazyb N. Diagnostic performance of sonoelastographic Tsukuba score and strain ratio in evaluation of breast masses. The Egyptian Journal of Radiology and Nuclear Medicine 49 (2018) 265-271.
171 Seo M, Ahn HS, Park SH, Lee JB, Choi BI, Sohn YM, Shin SY. Comparison andCombination ofStrain and ShearWave Elastography of Breast Masses for DifferentiationofBenign and Malignant Lesionsby Quantitative Assessment. J UltrasoundMed 2017; 00:00-00 | 0278-4297.
172 Zhao BX, Yao YJ, Zhou YC, Hao SY, Mu WJ. Strain Elastography: A Valuable Additional Method to BI-RADS? Published online: September 3, 2018 | Ultraschall in Med DOI https://doi.org/10.1055/s-0043-115108.
173 Mu WJl, Zhong WJl, Yao JYl, Li LJl, et al. Ultrasonic elastography research based on a multicenter study: adding strain ratio after 5-point scoring evaluation or not. PLoS ONE 2016;ll(2):e0148330. Feb 10.
174 Gheonea IA, Stoica Z, Bondari S. Differential diagnosis of breast lesions using ultrasound elastography. Indian J Radiol Imaging 2011;21(4):301-5.
175 Tardivon A, El Khoury, F. Thibault, C. Hardit. Elasto-echography of the breast. Journal de Radiologie 2006;87(10):1421.
176 Tardivon A, El Khoury, F. Thibault, C. Hardit. Elastography: techniques and results in breast pathology. Journal de radiologie 2008;89(10):Pages 1386-1387.
177 Kumm TR, Szabunio MM (2010) Elastography for the characterization of breast lesions: initial clinical experience. Cancer Control 17:156-161
178 . Chung EM, Cube R,Hall GJ et al. From the archives of the AFIP : breast masses in children and adolescents : radiologic-pathologic correlation. RadioGraphics, 2009, 29 : 907-931.
179 . Chao TC, Chao HH, Chen MF. Sonographic features of breast hamartomas. J Ultrasound Med, 2007, 26 : 447-452.
180 Tse GM, Law BK, Ma TK et al. Hamartoma of the breast: a clinicopathological review. J Clin Pathol, 2002, 55: 951-954.
181 Mutala TM, Ndaiga P, Aywak A. Comparison of qualitative and semiquantitative strain elastography in breast lesions for diagnostic accuracy. Cancer Imaging 2016; 16(2): 1-7.
182 Hatzung G, Grunwald S, Zygmunt M, Geaid AA, Behmdt PO, Isermann R, Kohlmann T, Ohlinger R. et al. Sonoelastography in the diagnosis of malignant and benign breast lesions: initial clinical experiences. Ultraschall Med. 2010 Dec; 31(6):596-603. doi: 10.1055/s- 0029-1245526. Epub 2010 Jul 7.
183 Hao SY, Jiang QC, Zhong WJ, et al. Ultrasound Elastography Combined With BI-RADS- US Classification System: Is It Helpful for the Diagnostic Performance of Conventional Ultrasonography? Clin Breast Cancer. 2016;16:e33-41.

184 Hao SY, Ou B, Li LJ, et al. Could ultrasonic elastography help the diagnosis of breast cancer with the usage of sonographic BIRADS classification? Eur J Radiol. 2015;84:2492- 500.
185 Zhi H, Xiao XY, Ou B, et al. Could ultrasonic elastography help the diagnosis of small (B2 cm) breast cancer with the usage of sonographic BI-RADS classification? Eur J Radiol. 2012;81:3216-21.
186 .Lee SH,Chung J, Choi HY, Choi SH, Ryu EB, Ko KH et al. Evaluation of Screening US-detected Breast Masses by Combined Use of Elastography and Color Doppler US with B- Mode US in Women with Dense Breasts: A Multicenter Prospective Study. Radiology. 2017 Nov;285(2):660-669.
187 Yi A, Cho N, Chang JM, et al. Sonoelastography for 1786 non-palpable breast masses: diagnostic value in the decision to biopsy. Eur Radiol 2012; 22:1033-40.
188 Tan SM, Teh HS, Mancer JF et al (2008) Improving B mode ultrasound evaluation of breast lesions with real-time ultrasound elastography - a clinical approach. Breast 17:252-257.
189 Cho N, Moon WK, Park JS et al (2008) Nonpalpable breast masses: evaluation by US elastography. Korean J Radiol 9:111-118.
190 Mohey N, Tamir A. Hassan. Value of mammography and combined grey scale ultrasound and ultrasound elastography in the differentiation of solid breast lesions. The Egyptian Journal of Radiology and Nuclear Medicine (2014) 45, 253-261.
191 Screening of breast lesions: a comparative study between mammography, B- mode ultrasonography, sonoelastography and histological results. Radiol Bras vol.46 no.4 São Paulo July/Aug. 2013.
192 Liu XJ, Zhu Y, Liu PF, Xu YL. Elastography for Breast Cancer Diagnosis: a Useful Tool for Small and BI-RADS 4 Lesions. *Asian Pacific Journal of Cancer Prevention, Vol 15, 2014.*
193 Fu LN, Wang Y, Wang Y, et al (2011). Value of ultrasound elastography in detecting small breast tumors. *Chin Med J,* **124,** 2384-6.
194 Engelken FJ, Sack I, Klatt D, et al (2012). Evaluation of tomosynthesis elastography in a breast-mimicking phantom. *Eur J Radiol,* **81,** 2169-73.
195 Carlsen JF, Pedersen MR, Ewertsen C, Sáftoiu A, Lönn L, Rafaelsen SR and Nielsen MB: A comparative study of strain and shear-wave elastography in an elasticity phantom. AJR Am J Roentgenol 204: W236-W242, 2015.
196 .Li L-J, Zeng H, Ou B, Luo B-M, Xiao X-Y, et al. (2014) Ultrasonic Elastography Features of Phyllodes Tumors of the Breast: A Clinical Research. PLoS ONE 9(1): e85257. doi:10.1371/joumal.pone. 0085257.
197 Kim GR, Choi JS, Han B-K, Ko EY, Ko ES, Hahn SY (2017) Combination of shear-wave elastography and color Doppler: Feasible method to avoid unnecessary breast excision of fibroepithelial lesions diagnosed by core needle biopsy. PLoS ONE 12(5): e017538.
198 Choi J, Koo JS. Comparative study of histological features between core needle biopsy and surgical excision in phyllodes tumor. Pathol Int. 2012; 62: 120-126. https://doi.Org/10.llll/i.1440-1827.2011. 02761.x PMID: 22243782.
199 Chang JM, Moon WK, Cho N et al. Clinical application of shear wave elastography (SWE) in the diagnosis of benign and malignant breast diseases. Breast Cancer Res Treat, 2011, 129:89-97.
200 Evans A, Whelehan P, Thomson K et al. Quantitative shear wave ultrasound elastography: initial experience in solid breast masses. Breast Cancer Res, 2010, 12:R104.
201 . Shin JY, Kim SM, Yun LB, Jang M, et al. Predictors of Invasive Breast Cancer in Patients With Ductal Carcinoma In Situ in Ultrasound-Guided Core Needle Biopsy. Journal of ultrasound in medicine. 2018, 10.1002/jum.l4722.
202 Bae JS, Chang JM, Lee SH, Shin SU, Moon WK. Prediction of inva- sive breast cancer using shear-wave elastography in patients with biopsy-confirmed ductal carcinoma in situ. Eur Radiol 2017; 27:7-15.
203 Cong R, Li J, Guo S. A new qualitative pattern classification of shear wave elastography for

solid breast mass evaluation. European Journal of Radiology 2017 ; Volume 87 , 111 - 119
204 . Berg WA, Mendelson EB, Cosgrove DO, et al. Quantitative Maximum Shear-Wave Stiffness of Breast Masses as a Predictor of Histopathologic Severity. Am J Roentgenol, 2015, 205:448-455
205 Evans, A. et al.Stiffness at shear-wave elastography and patient presentation predicts upgrade at surgery following an ultrasound-guided core biopsy diagnosis of ductal carcinoma in situ. Clinical Radiology ,2016, Volume 71 , Issue 11 , 1156 - 1159.
206 Lanigan, F., D. O'Connor, F. Martin, and W. M. Gallagher. 2007. Molecular links between mammary gland development and breast cancer. Cell Mol Life Sci 64:3159- 84.
207 Paszek, M. J., N. Zahir, K. R. Johnson, J. N. Lakins, G. I. Rozenberg, A. Gefen, C. A. Reinhart-King, S. S. Margulies, M. Dembo, D. Boettiger, D. A. Hammer, and V. M. Weaver. 2005. Tensional homeostasis and the malignant phenotype. Cancer Cell 8:241-54
208 Osuala KO, Sameni M, Shah S, et al. IL-6 signaling between ductal carcinoma in situ cells and carcinoma-associated fibroblasts mediates tumor cell growth and migration. BMC Cancer 2015 Aug 13;15:584. http://dx.doi.org/10.1186/sl2885-015-1576-3.
209 Martins D, Bee, a FF, Sousa B, et al. Loss of caveolin-1 and gain of MCT4 expression in the tumor stroma: key events in the progression from an in situ to an invasive breast carcinoma. Cell Cycle 2013 Aug 15;12(16):2684e90.
210 Vargas AC, McCart Reed AE, Waddell N, et al. Gene expression profiling of tumour epithelial and stromal compartments during breast cancer progression. Breast Cancer Res Treat 2012 Aug;135(l):153e65.
211 Quail DF, Joyce JA. Microenvironmental regulation of tumor progression and metastasis. Nat Med 2013; 19:1423-1437.
212 .Hao Y, Guo X, Ma B, Zhu L and Liu L. Relationship between ultrasound elastography and myofibroblast distribution in breast cancer and its clinical significance. Sci Rep 2016; 6: 19584.
213 Vargo-gogola et al, Nature Reviews cancer, 2007.
214 . Jin Y, Fenghua L, Jing D, Yifen G. Strain elastography features in invasive breast cancer: relationship between stiffness and pathological factors. Int J Clin Exp Med 2017;10(9):13290-13297.
215 Vinnicombe SJ, Whelehan P, Thomson K, McLean D, Purdie CA, Jordan LB, et al. What are the characteristics of breast cancers misclassified as benign by quantitative ultrasound shear wave elastography? *EurRadiol* 2014; 24: 921-6.
216 Brkljacic B, Divjak E, Tomasovic-Loncaric C, Tesic V, Ivanac G.*Shear-wave sonoelastographic features of invasive lobular breast cancers.* Croat Med J 2016, 57 (1). pp. 42-50.
217 Evans A, Whelehan P, Thomson K, McLean D, Brauer K, Purdie C, et al. Invasive breast cancer: relationship between shear-wave elastographic findings and histologic prognostic factors. Radiology. 2012;263(3):673-7.
218 Sim YT, Vinnicombe S, Whelehan P et al. Value of shear-wave elastography in the diagnosis of symptomatic invasive lobular breast cancer. Clin Radiol, 2015, 70;6; 604-609.
219 Grajo JR, Barr RG.Strain Elastography for Prediction of Breast Cancer Tumor Grades. Journal of ultrasound in medicine 2014; 33. 129-34. 10.7863/ultra.33.1.129.
220 .Christgen M, Steinemann D, Kuhnle E, *et al* Lobular breast cancer: clinical, molecular and morphological characteristics. Pathol Res Pract 2016; 212: 583-597-97.
221 Durhan G, Öztekin PS, Ünverdi H et al. Do Histopathological Features and Microcalcification Affect the Elasticity of Breast Cancer? J Ultrasound Med. 2017 Jun;36(6):1101-1108. doi: 10.7863/ultra. 16.06064. Epub 2017 Feb 27.
222 Chang JM, Park IA, Lee SH, Kim WH, Bae MS, Koo HR, et al. Stiffness of tumors measured by shear-wave elastography correlated with subtypes of breast cancer. Eur Radiol 2013;23(9):2450-8.

223 .Chen YL, Gao Y, ChangC et al. Ultrasound shear wave elastography ofbreast lesions: correlation of anisotropy with clinical and histopathological findings. Cancer Imaging (2018) 18:11
224 Acerbi I, Cassereau L, Dean I, Shi Q, Au A, Park C, et al. Human breast cancer invasion and aggression correlates with ECM stiffening and immune cell infiltration. Integrative Biology. 2015.
225 Levental KR, Yu H, Kass L et al (2009) Matrix crosslinking forces tumor progression by enhancing integrin signaling. Cell 139:891-906
226 Butcher DT, Alliston T, Weaver VM (2009) A tense situation: forcing tumour progression. Nat Rev Cancer 9:108-122
227 Lee SH, Moon WK, Cho N, Chang JM, Moon HG, Han W, Noh DY, Lee JC, Kim HC, Lee KB, Park IA. Shear-wave elastographic features ofbreast cancers: comparison with mechanical elasticity and histopathologic characteristics. Invest Radiol 2014; 49:147-155.
228 Youk JH, Gweon HM, Son EJ, Kim JA, Jeong J. Shear-wave elastography of invasive breast cancer: correlation between quantitative mean elasticity value and immunohistochemical profile. Breast Cancer Res Treat 2013; 138:119-126.
229 Ganau S, Andreu FJ, Escribano F, et al. Shear-wave elastography and immunohistochemical profiles in invasive breast cancer: evaluation of maximum and mean elasticity values. Eur J Radiol 2015; 84:617-622.
230 Hayashi M, Yamamoto Y et al. Associations Between Elastography Findings and Clinicopathological Factors in Breast Cancer. Medicine. 2015, 94(50): e2290.
231 .Denis M, Gregory A, Bayat M, Fazzio RT, Whaley DH, Ghosh K, Shah S, Fatemi M and Alizad A. Correlating Tumor Stiffness with Immuno histochemical Subtypes of Breast Cancers: prognostic value of Comb-Push ultrasound shear elastography for differentiating luminal subtypes. PLoS One 2016; 11: e0165003.
232 Romero Q, Bendahi, PO, Femö M, Grabau D and Borgquist S. A novel model for Ki67 assessment in breast cancer. *Diagn. Pathol.* **9,** 118 (2014).
233 Galant C, Berlière M, Leconte I, Marbaix E. New developments in histopronostic factors in breast cancer. Imagerie de la Femme (2010) 20, 9-17.
234 .Liu Y, Huang Y, Han J, Wang J et al. AssociationBetweenShearWave ElastographyofVirtual TouchTissue ImagingQuantificationParameters and theKi- 67ProliferationStatus in Luminal-TypeBreastCancer. J Ultrasound Med 2018; 00:00-00, 0278-4297.
235 Part A, Ellis MJ, Perou CM. Practical implications of gene-expression-based assays for breast oncologists. Nat Rev Clin Oncol 2011; 9 (1): 48-57._
236 Dominkovic MD, Ivanac G, Kelava T, Brkljacic B et al. Elastographic features of triple negative breast cancers Eur Radiol (2016) 26:1090-1097. DOI 10.1007/s00330-015-3925- 7.
237 . Wua T, Lib J, Wanga D, Lenga X, ZhangaL et al. Identification of a correlation between the sonographic appearance and molecular subtype of invasive breast cancer: A review of 311 cases. Clinical Imaging 53 (2019) 179-185.
238 . Wang D, Zhu K, Tian J, Li Z et al. Clinicopathological and Ultrasonic Features of TripleNegative Breast Cancers: A Comparison with Hormone Receptor-Positive/Human Epidermal Growth Factor Receptor-2-Negative Breast Cancers. J Ultrasound Med Biol, 2018 May;44(5): 1124-1132.
239 Li Z, Tian J, Wang X, Wang Y, Wang Z, Zhang L, Jing H, Wu T. Differences in multimodal ultrasound imaging between triple negative and non-triple negative breast cancer. Ultrasound Med Biol 2016; 42:882-890
240 Sohn YM, Seo M. Breast lesions diagnosed by ultrasound-guided core needle biopsy: Can shearwave elastography predict histologic upgrade after surgery or vacuum assisted excision?". Clinical Imaging 49 (2018) 150-155.
241 Chamming's F, Latorre-Ossa H, Le Frere-Belda MA, et al. Shear wave elastography of tumour growth in a human breast cancer model with pathological correlation. Eur Radiol 2013;

23:2079-2086.
242 Amaout-Alkarain A, Kahn AJ, Narod SA, Sun PA, Marks AN. Significance of lymph vessel invasion identified by the endothelial lymphatic marker D2-40 in node negative breast cancer. Mod Pathol 2007;20:183-91.
243 Pickup MW, Laklai H, Acerbi I, et al. Stromally derived lysyl oxidase promotes metastasis of transforming growth factor-betadeficient mouse mammary carcinomas. Cancer Res. 2013;73:5336- 5346.
244 Van Esser S, Veldhuis WB, van Hillegersberg R, van Diest PJ, Stapper G, ElOuamari M, et al. Accuracy of contrast-enhanced breast ultrasound for preoperative tumor size assessment in patients diagnosed with invasive ductal carcinoma of the breast. Cancer Imaging 2007;7:63-8.
245 Finlayson CA, MacDermott TA. Ultrasound can estimate the pathologic size of infiltrating ductal carcinoma. Arch Surg 2000;135(2): 158-9.
246 Allen SA, Cunliffe WJ, Gray J, Liston JE, Lunt LG, Webb LA, et al. Preoperative estimation of primary breast cancer size: a comparison of clinical assessment, mammography and ultrasound. Breast 2001;10(4):299-305.
247 Heusinger K, Lohberg C, Lux MP, Papadopoulos T, Imhoff K, Schulz-Wendtland R, et al. Assessment of breast cancer tumor size depends on method, histopathology and tumor size itself*. Breast Cancer Res Treat 2005;94(l): 17-23.

Appendix 1: Bi-Rads® ultrasound assessment categories

BI-RADS 0: Incomplete assessment, requiring further tests.

BI-RADS 1: Examination considered strictly normal

BI-RADS 2: Benign lesion(s): Simple cysts, intra-breast lymph nodes, breast implants, stable post-surgical changes, stable probable fibroadenomas.

BI-RADS 3: Anomaly probably benign. Suggestion of short-term surveillance. For example: solid masses with a circumscribed outline, oval, parallel orientation (probable fibroadenoma), complicated cysts that cannot be palpated, clusters of microcysts.

BI-RADS 4: Suspicious abnormality, with a probability of malignancy of between 2 and 95%, requiring histological analysis.

- 4a = low probability > 2% to < 10%,
- 4b = moderate probability > 10% to < 50%,
- 4c = high probability > 50 to < 95%.

BI-RADS 5: Highly suspicious abnormality with a probability of malignancy > 95%, requiring surgical removal.

BI-RADS 6: Known histological finding, proven malignancy

Appendix 2-1: Clinical information

Name :	First name :
Young filie's name: Age; I I I	Date of birth: I I| /I I |/I_I I I I №tel: I_U/U_I/LU_LLU

№ Examination date: IJJ I I I I I I_I LIJJJ Date:I_IJ/LI_I/LLLU

Clinical information

Weight(Kg) 1 1 1 1 Height (cm) I I I I	IMG I I I
Status genital activity □ AG+	□ AG - □ AG +/-
Age of menarchy I I I years	
age at menopause I_I_I years	
number of pregnancies / parity G I I / P II_I age of pregnancy I_I_I years	
breastfeeding □ no	□ yes Total duration I_I_I_I months
oral contraception □ non	□ yes Duration I_I_J years
hormone treatment□ no	□ yes Duration I I_I years
History	
Personal: breast cancer □ non	□ yes
undergoing radiotherapy or neoadjuvant chemotherapy for contralateral or neighbouring lesions	
□ no □ yes	
ovarian cancer □ no	□ yeswhen I I I_I I
Family: breast cancer □ no	□ yesage I_I_I years
□ grandmother □ mother□ sister	□ filie aunt□ □ cousin matemelle
ovarian cancer □ no	□ yes
Reason for consultation : □ screening □ pain	□ mass □ skin modification
□ nipple modification	□ axillary adenopathy
Evolution IIli months	
Coast : □ right breast □ left breast □ Bilateral	
Inspection	
Breast contours: □ normal□ curve	□ flat □ retraction
Skin changes: □ absence □ redness	□ thickening □ orange peel skin
Nipple changes: □ absence □ umbilication	□ retraction □ eczematiform erosion
Palpation □ absence of lesion □ placard□ nodule □ discharge	□ cederne cutaneous
If nodule: number I_I_I tarile N1I_I_I_I mm, N2I I I_I mm, N3 II_I I mm, N4 II_I mm, N5I_I_I_I mm	
siege □ QSE □ QIE □ QSI □ QII	□ UQS □ UQE □ UQInt □ UQInf
□ central □ axillary extension	□ sub mammary sillón
mobilile au plan superficie! aoui	□ no
deep mobilitò noui	□ no
Nodes: □ absent □ homolateral axillary hollow	□ sus claviculares □ contralateral axillary fossa

Appendix 2-2: examination

Nº d'examen : |_|_|_|_|_|_|_|_|_|_|_|_|_|_|_|
Date :|_|_|/|_|_|/|_|_|_|_|

Examen mammographique oui ☐ non ☐

Densité mammaire : ☐ a ☐ b ☐ c ☐ d

Côté : ☐ sein droit ☐ sein gauche

Masse : visible ☐ non ☐oui

taille M1|_|_|_| mm.

siège ☐ QSE ☐ QIE ☐ QSI ☐ QII ☐ UQS ☐ UQE ☐ UQInt ☐ UQInf

zone mammaire : ☐ antérieure ☐ moyenne ☐ postérieure

distance du mamelon |_|_|_|.|_|_|mm

Caractéristiques de la masse

Forme : ☐ ovale (elliptique, ovoïde) ☐ ronde (sphérique, globulaire) ☐ irrégulière

Contours : ☐ circonscrits ☐ masqués ☐ microlobulation ☐ indistincts ☐spiculés

Densité : ☐ hypodense ☐ isodense ☐ hyperdense ☐ calcique ☐ graisseuse

Signes associés ☐ non ☐ oui

☐ **Microcalcifications :** Nombre de foyer |_|_|

Distribution : ☐ segmentaire ☐ linéaire ☐amas ☐ régionale ☐ diffuses

Morphologie : ☐ rondes ou puctiformes ☐ amorphes ☐ grossières ou hétérogènes

☐ fines et pléomorphes ☐ fines linéaires ou branchées

☐ **Distorsion architecturale** ☐ **Asymétrie de densité** ☐ **Epaississement cutané**

☐ **Rétraction cutanée** ☐ **Rétraction mamelon** ☐**Ganglions axillaires**

Stade BI-RADS de l'ACR ☐ 0 ☐ 1 ☐ 2 ☐ 3 4 : ☐ a ☐ b ☐ c ☐ 5

Droit Sup. Gauche Sup. Droit Ext. Gauche Ext.

Appendix 2-3: Ultrasound examination

№ Examination date: |_|_|J_LLLLLLLLLI Date

Ultrasound examination

Echotexture Da Db □ c
Coast : □ right breast □ left breast
Mass :
seat QSE□ □ QIE DOSI üQII UQS UQE□ □ □ □ UQInf UQInthourly seat C1 П2 O3 П4 D5 O6 П7 08 П9 D10 D11 П12 size: LLLILIJtransversal x LLLI-LIJ height mm x J_| thickness mm.
major axis |_IJ_I |_|_| mm
distance to nipple |_|_|.|_|_| mm
distance from skin LLLIIJJ mm breast thickness |_|_|J.|_|_| mm
Mass characteristics
Shape : □ oval(macrolobulated)□ round□ irregular
Orientation : Lparallel to the skin □ not parallel to the skin

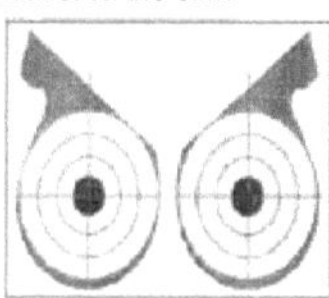

Contours :	L circumscnts o microlobulated□ indistinct□ angular□ spicules
Border :	□ fine□ hypoechoic halo
Echostructure :	□ anechogenic □ isoechoic □ hypoechoic
	□ hyperechoic D complex L heterogeneous

Posterior acoustic signs:□ no effect□ reinforcement□ attenuation□ combined
Calcifications:□ absent□ presentes□ in the mass□ outside a mass Vascularisation:□ absent□ present□ peripheral Li central□ peripheral and central Surrounding tissue;□ non□ architectural distortion□ echogenic galactophoric ectasia
□ skin thickening□ skin retraction□ nipple retraction
□ cedern□ hypervascularisation□ invasion of the pectoral muscle nodes : □ no□ yes
□ homolateral: axillary C□ central axillary□ sous claviculares
□ internal mammary□ supra clacivular
□ controlateral
BI-RADS stage of IACR ПO D1 C2 П3 4: Da Db Cc П5

Appendix 2-4: Elastographic examination

№ d'examen : LLLLLLLLLLLLIJ Date :|JJ/|JJ/LLLLI

Elastographic examination

Study of qualitative parameters

Homogeneity of cartography:□ homogeneous□ not very homogeneous□ heterogeneous
Maximum colour;□ red (soft component)□ green (intermediate component)□ blue (hard component)
Location of the hardest zone:□ intra-lesion□ peri-lesion □ intra and peri lesion
Presence of intra-lesional echo : □ presence □ echo void
Colorimetric score according to Itoh et al :
□1 C2 C3 П4 D5

Study of quantitative parameters

Elasticity ratio
Fat-Lésion Ratio (FLR)
Regions of interest (ROI) L of mass: LLIJ LIJ
Regions of interest (ROI) F subcutaneous fat tissue :
Ratio = F / L : |J_|J.|_|_|
Giande-Lésion Rapport (GLR)
Regions of interest (ROI) L of mass: LLLI LLI
Regions of interest (ROI) G adjacent glandular tissue: |_LU-LLI
Ratio = G/L:LUJU_I
Size ratio
Ratio = El / Ec : |LLI .| | |

Norn: First name :
Age ;|_|_| years

№ exam: LLLLLLLLLLLLLLI Date of sampling:| I |/| |_|/| |_|_|_I Date of report: I |_I/| I И I I I I

Side : □ right breast □ left breast
Type of sample amicrobiopsy □ macrobiopsy
Sampling topo □ QSE □ DIE □ QSI □ QII □ UQS □ UQE □ UQInt □ UQInf
□ central □ axillary prolon □ sub mammary sillón
Number of microscopic I |_I or macroscopic fragments collected I |_I

Microscopic examination

Benign lesions □ no □ yes

□ Adenofibroma □ Adenomyoepithelioma
□ Low-grade phyllodes tumour □ Papilloma
□ Fibrocystic masopathy. □ Other :

Malignant lesions □ no □ yes

□ carchoma in situ : □ ductal lobular □ □ mixed :
□ invasive carcinoma : □ NST □ lobular □ mixed:
□ other :
Histo-pronostic grade of SBR: □ 1 □ II □ III
Hormone receptors
CEstrogens : □ Positive □ Negative
Progesterones:□ Positive □ Negative
HER2 : □ Positive □ Negative
Ki67 : IJJ % (in French)
Molecular classification
□Luminal A. □ HER2
□Luminal B nTriple negative

Name First name :
Age; I I I years

Side : □ right breast □ left breast

Type of sampling□ lumpectomy□ lumpectomy / curage□ mastectomy / curage
Sampling chart OSE□ □ QIE QSI QII□ □ □ UQS UQE UQInt□ □ □ UQInf
□ centrai □ axillary extension or submammary sillón
Macroscopic lesion□ single□ 2 foci□ more than 2 foci Maximum distance between foci |J J J mm
Macroscopic size of the main lesion: |_I_U x LLIJ x Illi mm

Microscopic examination

Benign lesions □ no □ yes

□ Adenofibroma □ Adenomyoepithelioma

□ Low-grade phyllodes□ Papilloma

□ Fibrocystic mastopathy. □ Other :

Malignant lesions □ no □ yes

D caminóme in situ : □ ductal □ lobulare □ mixed :

□ caminóme Infiltrant : □ NST □ bbular□ mixed :

□ other :

Histoprognostic grade of SBR : □ 1 □ He □ III

Hormone receptors

CEstrogens:□ Positive □ Negative

Progesterones:□ Positive □ Negative

HER2 : □ Positive □ Negative

K¡67 : LU % % (IN %)

Molecular classification

□ Luminal A. □ HER2

□ Luminal B ^Triple negative

Vascular emboli □ absence□ presence Mucin: □ absence □ presence

Necrosis:□ absence □ presence

Sentinel lymph node □ no □ yes

Number of positive sentinel lymph nodes LU of which LU with isolated tumour cells

LLI with micrometastases LU with metastases

Lymph node removal □ no □ yes

Number of nodes sampled| 1 |

Number of positive nodes |J_J

of which LU with micrometastases LU with metastases

Appendix 3: Informed consent

Informed consent for ultrasound-guided breast biopsy ultrasound monitoring

A tissue fragment is removed using a needle for histological analysis.
This examination is carried out with your consent. You are free accept or refuse it.

How the exam works

You are seated and lying down in ultrasound room.
The radiologist uses ultrasound to identify the breast abnormality to be biopsied.
The skin is always disinfected and a local anaesthetic is administered, and a very small skin incision is made to allow the needle to be inserted painlessly.
The needle is guided on screen under ultrasound in the supine position, requiring you to remain perfectly still in order to guarantee millimetre-precision sampling.
The examination is not painful, but you will feel the sensation of movement in the breast.
You will hear a click as the needle moves inside the box during sampling.
The preparation time and the procedure last between 20 and 40 minutes.
A dressing is applied to the incision. This must be kept on for at least 24 hours.

The benefits of breast biopsy

The biopsy is used to check the nature of the anomaly detected. If the sample is sufficient, this procedure avoids the need for surgical biopsies under general anaesthetic to make the diagnosis, and also allows better planning of any surgery deemed necessary or specific breast monitoring.

Risks associated with biopsy

Any intervention on the human body, even when carried out under the most competent and safest conditions, carries a risk of complications.

- Biopsy involves risk of bleeding and/or haematoma, often with swelling, which usually resolves spontaneously.
- It is quite common for pain to be present at the biopsy site for up to 48 hours, and more rare for it to last longer.
- In very rare cases (less than 1%), infection or lesions of the skin or chest wall may occur.
- In exceptional cases, local anaesthesia may cause heart rhythm disorders or allergic reactions.

Questionnaire

Please answer following questions to avoid unnecessary risks. We can help you answer if you wish.

Do you have a blood disorder or frequent or prolonged bleeding (from the nose, for example)?	no □ yes □
Do you take blood-thinning drugs (Marcoumar®, Sintrom®, Heparin)?®	no □ yes □ If so, which ones?
Do you regularly take anti-platelet agents (Aspirin®, Plavix®, Ticlid®, etc....)?	no □ yes □ If so, which ones?
Are you allergic or intolerant to drugs, plasters, local anaesthetics or latex?	no □ yes □ If so, to what?
Do you suffer from any of the following illnesses?	
- Hypertension	no □ yes □
- Coagulation disorders	no □ yes □
- Serious heart disease	no □ yes □
- Diabetes	no □ yes □
Are you pregnant?	no □ ouin
Were you breastfeeding?	no □ yes □

Bring with you on the day of the exam

1. Your doctor's request (prescription, letter....).
2. **The results of the blood test** for coagulation and any other tests you may have been asked for.
3. The radiology file in your possession **(mammogram and breast ultrasound).**
4. **A written list of the medicines** you are taking.

For the exam

No hospitalisation is necessary and **you must not fast.**

I, the undersigned, having personally completed this form on
and gave my consent for the examination to be carried out.

Last name, First name Signature

Appendix 4: Glossary of statistical terms

1. Parameter of the diagnostic performance of a diagnostic test

	Disease present	No disease
Present sign	**A** VP (True Positives): these are affected individuals in whom the sign is present.	**B** FP (False Positives): the sign is present but the individuals are not affected.
Missing sign	**C** FN (False Negative): these are affected individuals in whom the sign is absent.	**D** VN (True Negative): the sign is absent and individuals are not affected.

2. Sensitivity

The sensitivity (Se) of a sign for a diagnosis is the probability that the sign is present in individuals affected by the disease under investigation, Se = A/ (A+C).

3. Specific

The specificity (Sp) of a sign for a diagnosis is the probability that the sign is absent in individuals not affected by the disease being investigated, Sp = D/(D+B).

4. Positive predictive value

The positive predictive value (PPV) of a sign for a diagnosis is the probability that the diagnosis is true if the sign is present, PPV = A/ (A+B).

5. Negative predictive value

The negative predictive value (NPV) of a sign for a diagnosis is the probability that the diagnosis will be false if the sign is absent, NPV = D/(C+D).

6. Accuracy

Accuracy (E) is obtained by dividing the correct responses (true positives + true negatives) by the total number of tests performed, E = (A+D) / (A+B+C+D).

7. False positive rate

The rate of false positives in healthy showing signs of the disease (B/A+B).

8. False negative rate

The rate of false negatives in sick individuals who do not show signs of the disease (C/C+D).

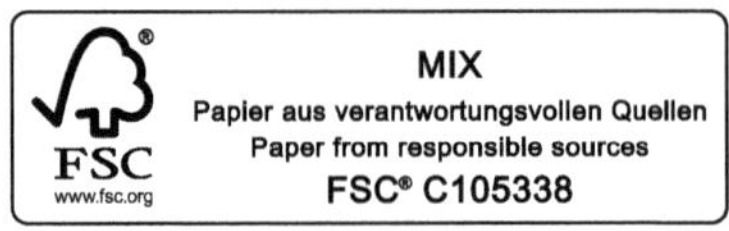

Printed by Books on Demand GmbH, Norderstedt / Germany